BASIC PUBLICATIONS USER'S GUIDE

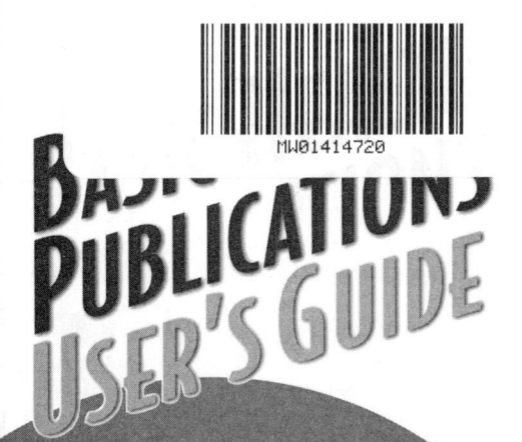

TO L-CARNITINE AND ACETYL-L-CARNITINE

Learn How to Use These Supplements to Boost Your Energy and Mental Focus.

VERA TWEED

JACK CHALLEM Series Editor

The information contained in this book is based upon the research and personal and professional experiences of the author. It is not intended as a substitute for consulting with your physician or other healthcare provider. Any attempt to diagnose and treat an illness should be done under the direction of a healthcare professional.

The publisher does not advocate the use of any particular healthcare protocol but believes the information in this book should be available to the public. The publisher and author are not responsible for any adverse effects or consequences resulting from the use of the suggestions, preparations, or procedures discussed in this book. Should the reader have any questions concerning the appropriateness of any procedures or preparations mentioned, the author and the publisher strongly suggest consulting a professional healthcare advisor.

Series Editor: Jack Challem
Editor: Karen Anspach
Typesetter: Gary A. Rosenberg
Series Cover Designer: Mike Stromberg

Basic Health Publications User's Guides are published by Basic Health Publications, Inc.
28812 Top of the World Drive
Laguna Beach, CA 92651
949-715-7327 • www.basichealthpub.com

Copyright © 2006 by Vera Tweed

ISBN-13: 978-1-59120-175-5
ISBN-10: 1-59120-175-6

All rights reserved. No part of this publication may be reproduced, stored in a retrieval system, or transmitted, in any form or by any means, electronic, mechanical, photocopying, recording, or otherwise, without the prior written consent of the copyright owner.

Printed in the United States of America

10 9 8 7 6 5 4 3 2

Contents

Introduction, 1

1. What Are L-Carnitine and Acetyl-L-Carnitine?, 3
2. Keeping the Heart Healthy, 10
3. Providing Energy for Exercise, 26
4. Enhancing Weight Loss, 42
5. Acetyl-L-Carnitine, Aging, and Mental Decline, 58
6. L-Carnitine, Acetyl-L-Carnitine, Diabetes, and Prediabetes, 63
7. Improving Male Fertility, 67
8. The Carnitine Program, 70

Conclusion, 73

Appendix A. Body Mass Index, 75

Appendix B. Low-Glycemic Foods, 78

Selected References, 80

Other Books and Resources, 85

Index, 87

Introduction

Energy is a precious commodity, not only in global oil markets but also in the human body. We need energy to stay alive, to do our jobs, to take care of ourselves and those we care about, and to work toward fulfilling our dreams. L-carnitine and acetyl-L-carnitine are supplements that are central to our body's ability to generate energy.

On the most basic level, L-carnitine enables the energy-producing component of our cells, the mitochondria, to do their jobs. The heart and skeletal muscles can't function optimally without it. With it, the heart can function at a much more efficient level. It isn't unrealistic to say that optimal supplies of L-carnitine could help to ward off a significant amount of the human suffering that comes about when the heart deteriorates. In the skeletal muscles, sufficient supplies of L-carnitine can relieve the fatigue that may discourage us from improving our health through regular exercise.

L-carnitine also has a pivotal role in weight management. Given that excess weight now affects the majority of the American population, is a precursor to the most common debilitating diseases, and can shorten our life span, any nutrient that can help with weight loss is extremely valuable.

Acetyl-L-carnitine is a specific form of L-carnitine that crosses the blood-brain barrier and can slow mental decline and aging. In addition, it reduces risk for diabetes and mitigates diabetic neuropathy, a life-threatening complication of the disease. And, among other benefits, a combination of L-carnitine and acetyl-L-carnitine improves male fertility.

Carnitine was identified a century ago, in 1905, as a nutrient in meat (*carnus* in Latin). Since then, it has become well established as an essential ingredient for optimum human health.

CHAPTER 1

WHAT ARE L-CARNITINE AND ACETYL-L-CARNITINE?

Carnitine is a nutrient that our bodies need to carry on the process of living. We get it from food, chiefly red meat and dairy products, and our livers make it, using other nutrients as building blocks: the amino acids lysine and methionine, iron, vitamins C and B_6, and niacin. While carnitine is the actual nutrient, L-carnitine is the bioavailable form that is found in supplements. In other words, L-carnitine is a form of the nutrient that our bodies can absorb and utilize. Once in our bodies, the nutrient itself is carnitine.

Because our bodies manufacture carnitine, the jury is out, medically speaking, on whether or not healthy people need to supplement with L-carnitine. In strict technical terms, it's considered a "conditionally essential nutrient," meaning that we need it if we're deficient, but no one has come up with a defined amount we should get on a daily basis. However, increasing evidence shows that many of us may suffer from less than optimal health or even disease because of insufficient carnitine in our bodies, caused by eating an inadequate diet or simply living longer.

Conditions that L-carnitine has helped to improve include:

- Aging
- Heart attack
- Heart failure
- Angina

User's Guide to L-Carnitine and Acetyl-L-Carnitine

- Diabetic neuropathy
- Insulin resistance
- Intermittent claudication
- Alzheimer's disease
- Parkinson's disease
- Muscle weakness
- Exercise-related fatigue
- Chronic fatigue syndrome and fibromyalgia
- Deficiency resulting from a vegetarian diet

The Common Denominator for Cellular Health

L-carnitine is linked to many conditions because we can't produce adequate energy to maintain cellular health without it. The chief food for the mitochondria in the heart and skeletal muscles is fat from our diet. L-carnitine acts as the cellular shipping and receiving system, delivering the fats (in the form of fatty acids) to the mitochondria to be burned for energy, and shipping out waste products.

> **Mitochondria**
> Long, thread-like structures that are the energy-producing parts of our cells. They are often referred to as the "powerhouses" of the cells.

This process must function efficiently for optimum health, but our mitochondrial function deteriorates as we age. L-carnitine supplementation has been found to arrest or reverse this decline and improve the function of the heart, skeletal muscles, brain, other organs, and overall cellular energy levels.

Severe Carnitine Deficiencies

Children are sometimes born with genetic disorders that prevent carnitine from being synthesized. They may suffer from a range of symptoms, including heart failure, muscle weakness, unexplained seizures, abnormal muscle tone or spasms,

What Are L-Carnitine and Acetyl-L-Carnitine?

blindness, deafness, dementia, stumbling, tremors, or cerebral palsy. Treatment, under medical supervision, may include prescription oral or intravenous supplementation with formulations of carnitine that are FDA-approved for use as a drug.

Among medical treatments, kidney dialysis is known to deplete carnitine. When carnitine is administered to dialysis patients—usually intravenously under medical supervision—side effects of extreme fatigue are markedly reduced. Some drugs used to treat cancer and HIV cause nerve damage, or neuropathy, which can be alleviated with medically supervised carnitine supplementation. Statin drugs, used to treat elevated cholesterol levels, deplete carnitine and CoQ_{10} levels. These supplements can alleviate muscle weakness, a common side effect, when they are used with statin therapy. The anticonvulsant medication, valproic acid, is also known to deplete carnitine.

Acetyl-L-Carnitine (ALC) and Other Forms of Carnitine

Acetyl-L-carnitine (ALC) is a form of carnitine developed for rapid absorption by the brain, as it crosses the blood-brain barrier. It is especially suitable for anyone who wants to enhance memory, learning, or concentration. Studies have shown that ALC may ward off Alzheimer's disease or other dementia, as well as improve mental function in healthy people. And, because ALC protects neurons in the brain and the central nervous system, it can also lessen peripheral nerve damage associated with diabetes.

> **Blood-Brain Barrier**
> *A selectively permeable protective membrane that controls whether substances in the blood can pass through into the brain tissue.*

Many studies of the role of carnitine in the treatment of heart disease have used another form of carnitine known as propionyl-L-carnitine

User's Guide to L-Carnitine and Acetyl-L-Carnitine

(PLC). This form was not available as a dietary supplement in the United States until recently, when a proprietary form of carnitine supplements, known as AminoCarnitines, became available. These contain the PLC form of the supplement.

The formulation of AminoCarnitines is based on scientific literature that shows that certain amino acids, such as glycine, arginine, and lysine, which are precursors to carnitine, improve the metabolic performance of the nutrient. When AminoCarnitines are manufactured, a proprietary, patented process is used to bind molecules of specific amino acids with L-carnitine in carefully controlled proportions. Consequently, each AminoCarnitine product always contains a consistent amount of the ingredients. When the supplement is taken, the bound molecules of amino acids and L-carnitine split apart in the intestinal tract, so both substances are available at the same time for maximum benefit. AminoCarnitine supplements are also available as Ester Carnitine.

In addition to ALC and AminoCarnitines, you will find the L-carnitine form and the L-tartrate and L-fumarate forms in supplements. The latter two are formulated with a base to facilitate absorption.

Who Needs L-Carnitine Supplements?

A significant body of research and clinical experience shows that L-carnitine, used with other nutrients that support heart function, can markedly improve the quality of life of people with heart disease. In some cases, patients waiting for a heart transplant who took the right combination of supplements, including L-carnitine, were able to restore heart function to a level where a transplant was no longer required.

Among healthy people, vegetarians may be deficient in carnitine because very little is supplied by their diet. Supplements can fill the gap.

What Are L-Carnitine and Acetyl-L-Carnitine?

TABLE 1.1. FOOD SOURCES OF CARNITINE

Food	Serving	Carnitine (mg)
Beef steak	3 ounces	81
Ground beef	3 ounces	80
Pork	3 ounces	24
Canadian bacon	3 ounces	20
Milk (whole)	8 fluid ounces (1 cup)	8
Fish (cod)	3 ounces	5
Chicken breast	3 ounces	3
Ice cream	4 ounces (1/2 cup)	3
Avocado	1 medium	2
American cheese	1 ounce	1
Whole-wheat bread	2 slices	0.2
Asparagus	6 spears (1/2 cup)	0.2

Athletes and people whose daily routine includes intense or extended exercise sessions can benefit from L-carnitine because it optimizes energy production and removes the toxic metabolites produced during intense activity that can cause pain or discomfort. Anyone who has difficulty exercising because of fatigue, shortness of breath, or poor circulation can benefit from L-carnitine's ability to increase the mitochondria's production of energy.

L-carnitine helps diabetics improve nerve function and manage blood glucose. And, for the millions of Americans who are at risk for diabetes because they suffer from insulin resistance (a condition also referred to as prediabetes or Syndrome X), the supplement can help improve insulin function. This same mechanism, along with L-carnitine's energy-enhancing action, may also help obese and overweight people lose weight.

Other conditions L-carnitine has helped improve include: male infertility, by improving the motility of sperm; nerve damage associated with HIV medications; early stages of age-related macular degeneration; and hyperthyroidism. Keep in mind that carnitine supplementation should be supervised by an appropriate qualified health professional when a medical condition is being treated.

How Safe Is Carnitine?

There are no known risks to taking any of the available forms of L-carnitine in dietary supplements. In 2004, a number of U.S. government agencies jointly sponsored *Carnitine: The Science Behind a Conditionally Essential Nutrient,* a major conference held at the National Institutes of Health campus in Bethesda, Maryland. The sponsoring agencies were the National Institute of Child Health and Human Development (NICHD), the National Center for Complementary and Alternative Medicine (NCCAM), the National Institute of Mental Health (NIMH), and the Office of Dietary Supplements (ODS). One of the conclusions from the conference: "Carnitine is a well-tolerated and generally safe therapeutic agent. No major negative/toxic effects were attributed to carnitine supplementation."

Getting Maximum Benefits from Supplementation

L-carnitine supplements will provide maximum benefits when they are part of a healthy lifestyle and, in some cases, work synergistically with other supplements. This User's Guide will provide the information you need to incorporate carnitine into your health routine. It includes information about relevant synergistic supplements that will increase the benefits derived from the carnitine supplementation, along with a review of the key elements of healthy living. It probably will not be surprising to note that the cornerstones in pre-

What Are L-Carnitine and Acetyl-L-Carnitine?

venting all of the major diseases that afflict our culture are exercise, a healthy diet, and weight management.

Exercise and weight loss are discussed at length because their effect is so far reaching in today's sedentary world. They are primary factors in the majority of diseases that pose the greatest threats to our health. This is where the benefits of L-carnitine excel, because carnitine supplementation helps users support higher levels of physical activity and makes it easier to stick to a healthy diet, metabolize food more efficiently, and have a leaner, healthier body. Most significantly, its benefits multiply when it is used to support, rather than substitute for, a good diet and exercise program.

The last chapter, The Carnitine Program, summarizes the key elements discussed in the Guide and provides recommended dosages for L-carnitine and related supplements.

CHAPTER 2

KEEPING THE HEART HEALTHY

Maintaining a healthy heart is probably the most important goal to work for when you are building a healthy lifestyle. Heart disease continues to be America's leading killer, the top reason for hospitalization, and the costliest disease to treat. In 2003, approximately two million people were hospitalized for heart attacks and heart conditions that can lead to a heart attack, such as blocked arteries. The cost for this care was $75 billion, according to the U.S. Agency for Healthcare Research and Quality, a government agency that tracks use and costs of healthcare services. Another 1.1 million people were hospitalized for congestive heart failure in that same year, at a cost of $26 billion.

Heart Conditions

The heart can malfunction in various ways. These problems and their causes are not fully understood, but the following list provides commonly used terms with descriptions of the conditions:

Atherosclerosis or Arteriosclerosis

Sclerosis means "hardening," in this case a hardening and thickening of the walls of the arteries. The process begins with plaque building up in the arteries, and can lead to a blockage of blood supply to the heart. That, in turn, can damage heart cells or cause a heart attack. There may be no visible symptoms of this condition until the arterial blockage is severe enough to cause chest pain, technically known as angina.

Angina Pectoris

This Latin term means "pain in the chest," or "pressure in the chest." When people experience an attack of angina, the symptoms are similar to a heart attack but, unlike the latter, they are temporary. In addition to chest pain, symptoms may include nausea, sweating, feeling lightheaded or dizzy, difficulty breathing, and pain in the throat, upper jaw, back, shoulder blades, or arms. Running to catch a bus, climbing stairs, or other physical exertion may prompt the symptoms, which can be terrifying. Although the pain and other manifestations subside with rest, immediate medical attention should be obtained to confirm the diagnosis and determine if treatment is necessary.

Myocardial Ischemia

Myocardial refers to the heart and *ischemia* means "not enough blood supply." Myocardial ischemia means the heart isn't getting enough blood, often because of atherosclerosis of one or more of the arteries that lead to the heart. Angina may or may not be a symptom.

Cardiomyopathy

This term is used to describe a heart that is too weak to pump blood properly to the rest of the body. This occurs because a key part of the heart, known as the left ventricle muscle, has weakened, and congestive heart failure can eventually result.

Myocardial Infarction

This is the technical term for a heart attack. It occurs after the heart has been significantly deprived of blood supply and, as a result, cells in one or more parts of the heart muscle have died. Symptoms are similar to angina, but rest doesn't bring relief.

Arrhythmia

The healthy heart beats with a steady rhythm, although it slows down when we sleep or rest and speeds up when we are more active. When its normal rhythm is disturbed, either by the heart beating too fast or too slow, the abnormal rhythm is called an arrhythmia. The cause may not be heart related but may be caused by lack of sleep, too much coffee, a fever, an overactive thyroid, or other factors. If it is a malfunction in the heart, however, it could be a sign of an electrical malfunction in the organ or narrowed arteries, due to plaque, that are limiting the heart's blood supply. Symptoms may include shortness of breath and fatigue, lightheadedness, panic sensations, or chest discomfort.

Congestive Heart Failure

When the heart cannot efficiently pump blood into or out of its chambers, fluid builds up in the lungs and heart. The lungs become stiff, resulting in shortness of breath, fatigue, and a constant sense of feeling weak, and the ankles or legs may swell. People with this condition may be woken up during the night by breathlessness, coughing or wheezing, and may experience frequent indigestion and a feeling of fullness.

Heart Failure

The early stages of heart failure do not produce congestion, but they are dangerous nevertheless. Consequently, the term "congestive" was dropped from the official name of this disorder in the recent guidelines issued jointly by the American College of Cardiology and the American Heart Association to differentiate it from the previous condition. In essence, the heart begins to fail while it still pumps normally, but it does not get an adequate supply of blood. There may be no seemingly dangerous symptoms such as shortness of breath at this stage, but the heart is abnormal, with changes in size or structure. The most common early symptoms of heart failure are fatigue and difficulty exercising, which may be incorrectly attributed to simply being out of shape or getting older.

The Mystery of Heart Failure

Heart failure is a progressive, rather than a sudden, occurrence. The heart gradually becomes less and less able to pump blood in and out of its chambers, and less able to pump adequate blood to other organs of the body. The risk of this condition is easy to overlook in these early stages because there are no dramatic, outward signs of deterioration. The American Heart Association estimates that five million people in the United States are affected by heart failure, and more than 550,000 cases are diagnosed annually.

Medical science has yet to fathom the causes of many cases of heart failure. In a British study of 100,000 cases of the disease, 39,000 cases were declared "idiopathic." However, L-carnitine and other, synergistic nutrients have demonstrated an ability to lessen or relieve this and other diseased states of the heart.

Idiopathic
A disease or condition that can't be traced to a known cause or origin.

When the heart functions, it obtains 60 percent of its energy from fatty acids. Without adequate carnitine, it isn't able to efficiently convert the fatty acids. It also needs carnitine to remove the toxic wastes that are a byproduct of the energy-production process.

In a study published in the journal *Clinical Cardiology* (among others), researchers at the University of Florida College of Medicine in Gainesville identified L-carnitine as one of the key substances that help the heart pump blood, even after a heart attack. They highlighted a multicenter trial of 472 patients who had suffered their first heart attack in their examination of the history of carnitine use among heart patients.

Patients were given either L-carnitine or a

placebo within twenty-four hours of the heart attack. For the first five days, the carnitine group received 9 grams of the nutrient per day intravenously, and then for twelve months, 6 grams daily of an oral L-carnitine supplement. Researchers measured the heart's ability to pump blood in and out to determine the results, and found that carnitine significantly improved this function. During the year-long study, 4 percent of the patients in the carnitine group experienced heart failure, compared with 10 percent in the placebo group.

Surviving a Heart Attack

Several studies have shown that fewer people die after a heart attack if they take L-carnitine. In one twelve-month study of 160 people who had suffered a heart attack, half were given 4 grams of L-carnitine and the other half received a placebo. All the patients continued to take prescribed medication. By the end of the year-long trial, 1.2 percent of those taking carnitine had died, compared to 12.5 percent of those taking the placebo.

Another study examined the effect of L-carnitine supplementation for twenty-eight days on 100 patients who experienced symptoms of a heart attack. The double-blind study divided patients into two groups, those taking 2 grams of L-carnitine daily and those taking a placebo. In the carnitine group, 15 percent of the patients died, compared to 26 percent of patients in the placebo group.

Improving Quality of Life

Other studies have looked at patients' quality of life once heart disease has developed. Healthy people take their ability to perform the usual tasks of daily living for granted, from taking a shower or making the bed in the morning to walking around the office or shopping in a supermarket and putting the groceries away. However, anyone whose heart function is compromised may not be able to carry out such seemingly mundane tasks. The required effort exceeds their energy levels and may lead to extreme fatigue, chest pain, or other discomfort.

One key way in which L-carnitine's impact has been measured is to examine the effect of the supplement on heart patients' ability to exercise. Researchers have been able to quantify and compare improvement in the ability of the heart to do its job by using measures such as treadmill or bicycle stress tests, which are much more physically demanding than routine day-to-day activities. Such studies of people with angina or other heart malfunctions have been carried out for more than twenty years, and have shown that carnitine significantly improves heart function and, consequently, the quality of life. These are some of the studies:

- In 1984, Japanese researchers examined the impact of L-carnitine on twelve patients with stable angina pectoris. In this multistage study, published in the *Japanese Heart Journal*, researchers first gave participants a placebo and performed treadmill stress tests. Then all twelve people took 900 milligrams of L-carnitine daily, and treadmill stress tests were performed after four and twelve weeks of supplementation. The impressive results of this small study: two patients were completely free of angina after taking L-carnitine, and all were able to exercise on the treadmill significantly longer after L-carnitine supplementation.

- In 1985, researchers in Italy investigated the effect of L-carnitine on forty-four men with stable chronic angina in a multicenter, double-blind, randomized, placebo-controlled crossover trial. In this study, published in the *International Journal of Clinical Pharmacology, Therapy and Toxicology*, subjects took either a placebo or 1 gram of L-carnitine twice daily. Their ability to exercise on a stationary bicycle was measured in terms of how much effort they could expend before experiencing symptoms of angina. After taking L-carnitine for four weeks, 23 percent of the men ceased to experience angina, and all were able to cycle at a higher intensity when taking the L-carnitine than when taking a placebo.

- In 1991, another Italian study at three centers examined 200 patients between the ages of forty and sixty-five who were being treated with medication for exercise-induced angina. In this study, published in the journal *Drugs Under Experimental and Clinical Research,* 100 patients were randomly selected to take 2 grams of L-carnitine daily in addition to their usual medications. When the exercise ability of the carnitine group was compared to those not taking the supplement, researchers found that L-carnitine improved the function of the heart both during exercise and at rest, and also improved cholesterol levels. In some cases, less medication was required as patients ceased to experience undue fatigue, difficulty breathing, or palpitations in the course of normal daily activity.

- In 1998, researchers at the Veteran's Administration Medical Center in Minneapolis, Minnesota, examined the effect of L-carnitine on thirty patients with chronic congestive heart failure in a single-blind, randomized, placebo-controlled study published in the journal *Cardiovascular Drugs and Therapy*. Subjects received a single intravenous dose of propionyl-L-carnitine (a form of the supplement that will be discussed in-depth later on), and 1.5 grams of the supplement in oral form daily for one month. After fifteen days, patients taking the supplement experienced improvement in pulmonary arterial pressure and exercise capacity, with 21-percent improvement in the time they could exercise, and improvements in heart structure and function. Improvement in quality of life was significant, given that this group experienced fatigue, palpitations, or difficulty breathing with small amounts of physical activity.

- In 2000, researchers in India tested L-carnitine on forty-seven people with chronic stable angina. In this study, published in *The Journal of the Association of Physicians of India*, participants received either 2 grams daily of L-carnitine or a placebo. Computerized stress tests measured their ability to exercise, including duration and time to recover, at the beginning of the study and after three months of supplementation. Those taking L-carnitine significantly improved the length of time they were able to exercise and the recovery time after exercise, while no improvement was seen among those taking a placebo.

Synergy with CoQ$_{10}$

These studies show that L-carnitine, by itself, can provide substantial improvement for people suffering from various aspects of heart disease. It is important to study the role of individual nutrients in research settings to learn about their impact on human health, but in clinical settings, enhancing the well-being of the patient is the objective. Nutritionally oriented physicians are therefore likely to use L-carnitine with other supplements for a synergistic effect.

Synergy
The ability for one substance to enhance the actions of another substance.

Cells in our bodies do not use individual nutrients in isolation, and in some cases, a certain combination of nutrients is particularly beneficial

User's Guide to L-Carnitine and Acetyl-L-Carnitine

because of the interplay of their mechanisms. Such is the relationship between L-carnitine and Coenzyme Q_{10}, commonly referred to as CoQ_{10}.

As mentioned earlier, carnitine is the transport system that shuttles fatty acids into the energy-generating mitochondria in the cells of the heart. Once the fatty acids have been delivered, CoQ_{10} acts as the spark plug that turns the fats into energy. This energy is produced in the form of ATP, or adenosine triphosphate. ATP is considered the energy of life because our bodies use ATP molecules as energy to carry on the process of living.

> **ATP**
> Adenosine triphosphate, the energy molecule our bodies use as fuel to sustain life.

To stay alive, we have to continually manufacture ATP. We have only about 700 milligrams of ATP in the body at any one time, which is enough for about ten heartbeats. It is estimated that our hearts beat approximately 86,000 times in the course of a day.

The cycle of ATP being created and used, created and used, created and used goes on continually when everything is functioning as it should. Efficient production of ATP is synonymous with good health. Conversely, a malfunction in the process is the beginning of a slippery slope toward diseased states. The cycle of ATP production breaks down without adequate CoQ_{10} as well as carnitine.

Studies performed in the past few decades give us a sense of the powerful role of CoQ_{10} in the function of our hearts. Forty-one controlled human trials between 1972 and 2005 found that CoQ_{10} provided a benefit. These are the findings of some of this research:

- A study published in 1992 in *Biochemical and Biophysical Research Communications* noted that there were 20,000 patients in the United States eligible for heart transplants, but less than one-tenth of that number of donors available. Eleven transplant candidates were treated with CoQ_{10} and all experienced significant improvement. Some patients required no medication and had no limitation or discomfort related to normal physical activity after taking CoQ_{10}.

- In 1993, a double-blind, placebo-controlled trial of 641 people suffering from congestive heart failure was published in *The Clinical Investigator*. In addition to medications they were already taking, participants took either a placebo or CoQ_{10} for one year, at a dosage of 2 milligrams per kilogram of body weight. There were 20 percent fewer hospitalizations and less than half the number of instances of pulmonary edema or cardiac asthma in the CoQ_{10} group than there were in the placebo group.

- A double-blind, placebo-controlled study published in 1998 in *Cardiovascular Drugs and Therapy* tested the ability of CoQ_{10} to help patients regain health after a heart attack. In the study of 144 patients, half took 120 milligrams of CoQ_{10} daily while the rest took a placebo, and both groups were monitored for twenty-eight days. Among the CoQ_{10} group, incidence of angina pectoris and disturbed heart rhythm was approximately one-third of that in the placebo group. CoQ_{10} also improved the condition of the structure of the heart.

- In 2003, a similar but longer-term study of the effect of CoQ_{10} after heart attack was published in *Molecular and Cellular Biochemistry*. A group of 144 cardiac patients took either 120 milligrams per day of CoQ_{10} or placebo for one year. During that time, the placebo group suffered approximately twice the number of non-fatal heart attacks as the CoQ_{10} group. Also, levels of HDL (the "good" cholesterol)

User's Guide to L-Carnitine and Acetyl-L-Carnitine

increased significantly among those taking CoQ_{10}.

- In 2004, a study published in *Clinical Cardiology* reinforced earlier findings about the benefits of CoQ_{10} for patients awaiting a heart transplant. Researchers in Israel noted that the number of people needing a heart transplant was increasing faster than available donors. They randomly selected thirty-two patients with end-stage heart failure. They gave half of these patients a special preparation of CoQ_{10} designed to be absorbed especially well through the intestine, and a placebo to the other half. All of the patients continued their usual conventional treatment. After three months, the patients taking CoQ_{10} were able to walk and breathe better and generally function better in their normal lives.

Synergy with D-Ribose

Stephen Sinatra, M.D., a board certified cardiologist who is a pioneer in the use of nutritional therapy for treating heart and other diseases, has used the combination of CoQ_{10} and L-carnitine in his practice for many years. Recently he identified a third nutrient that works in synergy with CoQ_{10} and L-carnitine, both to restore heart function and to prevent disease from developing: D-ribose (also called ribose).

When the heart pumps blood, each heartbeat has two critical phases: The heart relaxes to allow blood to enter its chambers in what is technically called the diastolic phase. Then it contracts, which pushes the blood out, in what is known as the systolic phase. An adequate supply of ATP, the body's energy molecule, is mandatory for this process.

Diastolic Function
The action of the heart when it relaxes to take in blood during each heartbeat.

D-ribose improves the diastolic, or relaxation,

phase of the cycle and restores the supply of ATP. Clinical research has shown that these benefits occur in people with heart disease and in healthy, exercising people. In other words, D-ribose dramatically improves the heart's recovery time after exercise or any strenuous exertion.

> **Systolic Function**
> *The action of the heart when it contracts to eject blood during each heartbeat.*

The study of D-ribose began in Japan in 1944, and numerous studies since then have examined its role in the function of the heart. When the supply of blood to the heart is inadequate, as is the case in ischemia, the replenishment of energy—ATP—has a time lag. Consequently, when patients with ischemia do treadmill stress tests as part of their medical checkups, they routinely experience extreme fatigue after the exertion and may take days or longer to recover.

In a German study published in the *Lancet* in 1992, researchers tested ribose on twenty men with severe coronary artery disease that resulted in 75 percent or greater narrowing in at least one blood vessel. In a double-blind trial, they gave the men either a placebo or an oral supplement containing 15 grams of ribose four times daily for three days. They gave the men exercise stress tests on the fifth day after beginning the protocol, and found that those who had taken ribose were able to exercise significantly longer than the placebo group before they experienced shortness of breath.

Another German study, published in the *European Journal of Heart Failure* in 2003, examined the impact of ribose on fifteen patients with congestive heart failure. The study was double-blind and placebo-controlled, and used a crossover method, in which patients were divided into two groups. Each group took either placebo or ribose for three weeks using a dosage of 5 grams of

D-ribose three times daily, then had a one-week wash-out period, then switched substances for three weeks. Researchers then tested subjects on a stationary bicycle and used a questionnaire to assess changes in quality of life. They found that the D-ribose significantly increased the amount of blood flow to the heart and improved physical function and quality of life.

Metabolic Cardiology

L-carnitine, CoQ$_{10}$, and D-ribose make up a synergistic trio of nutrients that are part of what Sinatra calls metabolic cardiology. Ultimately, the trio works to optimize the production of ATP, the energy without which a human body cannot survive, and which directly decreases optimal function when its production is compromised. He explains his theory and treatment fully in his book, *The Sinatra Solution* (Basic Health, 2005).

Mitochondrial health is the cornerstone of metabolic cardiology. Although mitochondria are present in cells throughout the body, there are far more of them in the heart. According to Sinatra, you might have 200 mitochondria per cell in your bicep, but 5,000 mitochondria per cell in your heart. In fact, about one-third of the heart is composed of mitochondria, making the health of this component of cells paramount in importance.

Focusing on mitochondrial health and improving ATP production can make dramatic differences in the quality of life of people with heart disease. In Sinatra's practice, where he routinely uses exercise stress tests as a normal part of evaluation of patients' health status, shortness of breath generally goes away within a few minutes after such tests. However, a common complaint from patients is: "I was exhausted for a week." Consequently, heart patients are often reluctant to receive a stress test, even though it's a necessary part of monitoring their status.

Keeping the Heart Healthy

"I never understood why [this occurred]," says Sinatra. However, through years of research and practice, he has been able to solve the riddle. "When you have a diseased heart," he explains, "you're leaking ATP; it's almost like taking a pail of water and putting a few holes in it." By taking the therapeutic trio—L-carnitine, CoQ$_{10}$, and D-ribose—Sinatra's patients are able to perform their stress tests without the aftereffect of debilitating fatigue and their ability to function in everyday life is significantly improved.

The Challenge of Preventing Problems

The heart is an incredibly efficient, hardworking organ. Take your own pulse and count the beats. Then, imagine clenching your fist that many times per minute, and doing it twenty-four hours a day, seven days a week, throughout your entire life. And keep in mind that the heart keeps pace as your activity levels change from sleeping to moderate movement to more intense activity, pumping the needed amount of blood to the your body no matter what else is going on. That's if it's working as it should.

Part of the problem of keeping your heart in shape is that, despite its almost miraculous ability to do the job nature has given it, the heart is not very good at letting you know when there's a slight problem. It doesn't have a sophisticated warning mechanism like some of today's cars, which can tell you if the air pressure in a tire is slightly down. It doesn't even have the most elemental indicator of fuel (ATP), like a gas gauge that monitors amount of fuel and its usage mile by mile.

It's almost as though the heart was constructed with the idea that nothing could ever go wrong, or perhaps it was given such a sophisticated role that there was no way to build in an error-detection system as well. The heart doesn't even have nerves that feel pain directly. When people feel pain during a heart attack, it's because nerves in the heart short-circuit other nerves, which then communicate pain. That's part of the reason why heart attack symptoms can be so varied, and why it is so difficult to recognize problems before they develop into serious disease.

Getting a Head Start on Heart Health

Given that slight malfunctions are practically undetectable in our daily lives, it's easy to adopt the perspective that "no news is good news," and pay no attention to our heart. So, perhaps it's not surprising that the most common heart-related symptom likely to make a person visit his or her doctor is shortness of breath. However, this isn't the first thing that has gone awry with the heart.

Remember, when the heart beats and pumps blood, it has two basic actions: relaxing to take in blood (diastolic function), and contracting to eject blood (systolic function). By the time a person notices that they're short of breath—certainly if the condition has become so noticeable that he or she steps into a doctor's office—the heart is not contracting as it should, or not ejecting blood optimally. Unfortunately, that's a sign that malfunction has progressed beyond the first stage.

Before the heart has difficulty ejecting blood by contracting, its action of relaxing and taking in blood may not have been operating properly for some years. In other words, the breakdown of diastolic function is at a more advanced stage. It may have begun years before the person started chasing his or her grandchild and suddenly stopped short, feeling very out of breath.

Sinatra estimates that 60 to 70 million Americans have diastolic dysfunction and a lot of them are not aware of it. Nature is not about to add a sensitive error-detection system from luxury car manufacturers to detect decreases in your heart's

Keeping the Heart Healthy

ability to fully relax with each heart beat, so what can you do?

Protect yourself. Add the trio of L-carnitine, CoQ$_{10}$, and D-ribose to your regular routine of daily supplements. They serve multiple functions: L-carnitine shuttles fatty acids into the mitochondria and removes waste products; CoQ$_{10}$ sparks the furnace to burn the fats; and D-ribose promotes the production of energy in the form of ATP, the energy molecule your heart thrives on. The trio also has antioxidant properties, so these nutrients help to prevent free radicals from damaging your heart. Add magnesium to your daily regimen. This mineral helps your heart perform that crucial relaxation phase of each heartbeat.

In addition to taking the right dietary supplements, maintaining a strong heart also requires a healthy diet, weight management, and exercise. L-carnitine can help with all of these.

> **Free Radicals**
>
> *A product of normal cell metabolism, these atoms or molecules have an unpaired electron that tries to grab an electron from a complete molecule. The resulting damage is a factor in aging, arterial plaque, and a number of degenerative diseases including heart disease.*

CHAPTER 3

PROVIDING ENERGY FOR EXERCISE

When you go to the doctor for a routine physical exam, your fitness level will most likely not be tested if you're relatively healthy. In fact, your doctor may not even ask you about your exercise habits. However, your fitness level is a key indicator of your health, your likelihood of developing the debilitating diseases that plague our culture, and your potential life span. Some members of the medical profession are encouraging their peers to start tracking your exercise habits—or lack of exercise—for this reason.

Researchers from the Division of Cardiovascular Medicine at Duke University Medical Center in Durham, North Carolina, recently noted in the *New England Journal of Medicine:* "Exercise testing is routinely used to evaluate patients with symptoms," but is not currently used to evaluate healthy people. They went on to say that cardiorespiratory fitness (how intensely and how long our heart allows us to exercise) "provides strong and independent prognostic information about the overall risk of illness and death, especially that from cardiovascular causes."

The correlation between fitness and health relates to a wide range of conditions in both men and women. "It is valid in apparently healthy persons;" stated the experts from Duke University, "in patients with a broad range of maladies, including several types of cancer and cardiovascular disease; and in at-risk patients with diabetes mellitus, the metabolic syndrome, and hypertension." Consequently, they are asking the medical community to take note and put this knowledge to use: "We hope that this report will provide a stimulus to reintroduce fitness assessments into the routine clinical environment for both women and men."

The American College of Sports Medicine and the Centers for Disease Control and Prevention recommend thirty minutes of at least moderate exercise on all or most days of the week. A decade ago, research showed that following these recommendations reduced the risk of death from cardiovascular disease by half.

How Fitness Levels Decline as We Age

As we age, on average, it's estimated that our cardiorespiratory fitness declines by one percent per year. If you're about to celebrate your fortieth or fiftieth birthday and think, "Gee, I'll be one percent less fit," that thought may not seem too alarming, but small decreases in your heart's capacity add up, and this decline accelerates as we live longer.

The Baltimore Longitudinal Study of Aging tracked 375 men and 435 women between the ages of twenty-one and eighty-seven, who were all in good health, and periodically tested their fitness levels on treadmills. To quantify aerobic capacity, researchers used a measure that is considered a standard in the medical and fitness communities: the amount of oxygen the body consumes during exercise, technically known as VO2. The underlying premise is that as aerobic capacity diminishes a person commonly does less physical activity, walks slower, and becomes exhausted with physical exertion more easily.

Aerobic Exercise
Activity that makes the heart work harder, increasing heart rate and strengthening the heart muscle in the process.

The study, published in the American Heart Association journal, *Circulation*, found that aerobic capacity declines at a significantly greater rate as we live longer: by 3 to 6 percent per decade in our twenties and thirties, but by 20 percent or more per decade in our seventies and beyond.

This is how the lead author of the study, Jerome Fleg, M.D., a cardiologist and medical officer in the Division of Epidemiology and Clinical Applications at the National Heart, Lung, and Blood Institute in Bethesda, MD, put these findings in perspective: "The rate of decline in the population-at-large is probably somewhat greater than what we observed here, because many older people will have disease-related deficits in addition to those brought on by age."

There is a positive side to these results, however. "Over time, your aerobic capacity will decline, but at any given age someone who exercises will have a higher capacity than someone who is a couch potato," said Fleg. "By participating in a training program, you can raise your aerobic capacity 15 percent to 25 percent, which in our study would be equivalent to being ten to twenty years younger." In addition to aerobic exercise, he recommends resistance or weight training: "Declining muscle strength, another factor that contributes to frailty as people age, can also be countered through strengthening exercises."

How Exercise Benefits Our Health

We know that L-carnitine supplementation improves cardiovascular health, but it isn't designed to replace exercise. In fact, it can help your body produce energy more efficiently, so exercise is easier, and it can help your heart and other muscles recover more rapidly after your exercise routine.

When you do aerobic exercise you breathe faster and more deeply to increase the amount of oxygen in your bloodstream. Small blood vessels dilate to get more oxygen to your muscles, and

Providing Energy for Exercise

they also carry away waste products. With regular exercise your muscles actually develop more blood vessels to deliver more oxygen and remove waste products more efficiently. Your whole body functions more efficiently.

The most important thing about exercise is to do it regularly. The type of exercise you do and the length of each workout is less important; it's the consistency that counts more than anything else. Key benefits of physical activity include increased cardiovascular health, reduced risk of stroke, as well as lowered hypertension, unhealthy cholesterol levels and type 2 diabetes, but there are many other perks. Exercise certainly helps in maintaining a healthy weight. Here is a list of some of the things we know, from scientific studies, about how regular exercise can improve your health and the quality of your life, at any age:

Resistance Training
Exercise that strengthens and builds muscles by using weights or some other type of resistance.

- People who exercise are likely to be more productive at work, are less likely to become stressed by work situations, find greater enjoyment in their jobs, and are less likely to get tired in the afternoon.

- Inflammation, a precursor to virtually all major debilitating diseases, including heart disease, diabetes, and cancer, can be measured with a blood test known as a C-reactive protein (CRP) test. People who get moderate exercise regularly are 15 percent less likely to have unhealthy, elevated levels of CRP, and those who exercise regularly with vigorous workouts are 47 percent less likely to have elevated CRP levels.

- Physical activity lowers the risk of reduced bone mass, known as ostopenia; reduced bone mineral density, or osteoporosis; and sarcopenia, the technical term for reduced muscle mass as a result of aging. Sarcopenia manifests itself as frailty among the elderly and can severely limit a person's ability to function, because strength is lost as muscle mass decreases, and normal tasks such as walking or taking a shower can become difficult.

- Exercise eases depression. In a group of people who suffered mild to moderate depression, symptoms were reduced by 50 percent by doing thirty-minute sessions of aerobic exercise three times per week.

- Research with animals shows that exercise slows the development of small changes in the brain that eventually lead to Alzheimer's disease.

- People who suffer from chronic low back pain can get relief with exercise. Studies that examined a total of 6,000 people showed that, contrary to earlier theories promoting rest for relief of low back pain, exercise is better.

- Exercise can improve your sex life, both mentally, by enhancing mood and self-esteem, and physically, by improving blood flow throughout your body.

- Older people who exercise may suffer fewer hip fractures because their bones may be better able to withstand force.

Most people don't get enough exercise despite the overwhelming evidence in its favor. According to figures compiled by the Centers for Disease Control and Prevention, the percentage of Americans who get no leisure-time physical activity has decreased during recent years, from 32 percent in 1996 to 25 percent in 2002. However, other estimates show that most Americans are still not getting at least thirty minutes of exercise most days of the week, the minimum amount recommended for good health.

Providing Energy for Exercise

Overcoming the Serious Challenges to Your Exercise Routine

There is an endless list of possible excuses for not getting regular exercise or, at least for not being more active during the course of the day. Lack of energy can be viewed as an excuse, but for many people it's a debilitating reality, not simply a justification for inactivity. This is particularly true for people who suffer from heart disease and, as a result, experience shortness of breath, chest pain, or extreme fatigue upon even mild exertion. Supplementing with L-carnitine can definitely help in these cases, as shown by the studies in the previous chapter. Other conditions show equal improvement with supplementation.

Peripheral Arterial Disease

Another debilitating condition that can make walking very arduous if not impossible is peripheral arterial disease, or intermittent claudication, which is caused by poor circulation in the legs. L-carnitine can significantly help in such situations. There are numerous studies demonstrating such a benefit, including the following, both published in 2001:

- Australian researchers, writing in *Medicine and Science in Sports and Exercise*, reported that propionyl-L-carnitine, a specific form of L-carnitine, improved walking performance among people with peripheral arterial disease, in which walking is painful. The researchers compared the walking ability of the participants while taking a placebo or L-carnitine, and found that walking distance improved and calf muscle strength increased significantly after four weeks of supplementation.

- Researchers at the University of Colorado Health Sciences Center in Denver reported findings from a double-blind, placebo-controlled study of 155 patients in the *American Journal of Medicine*. Seventy-two of the patients were located in the United States and eighty-three were in Russia. All had disabling claudication that impaired their walking ability. During the six-month trial, participants received either a placebo or 2 grams daily of propionyl-L-carnitine. At the outset, and after three and six months, the subjects were evaluated on a treadmill moving at two miles per hour with an incline of 0 percent, which was increased in increments of two percent every 2 minutes until symptoms of claudication prevented them from walking further. At the six-month mark, L-carnitine had increased walking time by 54 percent and reduced physical pain. A questionnaire filled in by participants indicated L-carnitine significantly improved their ability to function in daily life.

Kidney Disease

Another condition that results in debilitating fatigue is kidney failure, which requires dialysis treatments. Carnitine supplies are depleted during the treatment, leaving patients with very low levels of energy. Replenishing carnitine can improve their energy levels, as this study shows:

- At Harbor University of California at Los Angeles Medical Center in Torrance, researchers examined the impact of intravenous L-carnitine on the ability of dialysis patients to exercise, as such patients typically experience debilitating fatigue. In two randomized, placebo-controlled trials, published in 2001 in the *American Journal of Kidney Diseases*, a total of sixty patients received either L-carnitine or a placebo three times a week for twenty-four weeks, following their dialysis treatments. After testing the patients' oxygen capacity and administering questionnaires to determine changes in quality

Providing Energy for Exercise

of life, the researchers concluded: "Intravenous L-carnitine treatment increased plasma carnitine concentrations, improved patient-assessed fatigue, and may prevent the decline in peak exercise capacity in hemodialysis patients."

How L-Carnitine Can Help Everyone

Most of us face far less formidable energy challenges, but even these can present major stumbling blocks to formal exercise or simply walking a few extra blocks instead of driving. Because L-carnitine can help our bodies produce energy more efficiently, it may give us an extra boost that will make a morning, lunchtime, or evening workout or a weekend hike a pleasant experience. It can also help serious athletes recover from grueling training.

There are two key areas of the body where carnitine does its work: the heart (as described in the previous chapter) and in skeletal muscle. In skeletal muscles, carnitine increases the efficiency of energy generation and, equally important, toxin removal. It also acts as an antioxidant, which is important during exercise, since increased activity causes greater production of free radicals.

Many fitness trainers and sports nutritionists recommend taking L-carnitine to improve recovery from intense exercise. For example, Rehan Jalali, author of *The Six-Pack Diet Plan*, (Basic Health, 2005), is a specialist in nutrition for athletes. He has worked with physicians who specialize in sports medicine and clients who must meet exceptionally high fitness standards. He recommends taking 1 to 2 grams of a liquid form of L-carnitine one hour before a training session.

These are some of the studies that have examined the action of L-carnitine in exercise:

- In a study published in 1990 in the *International Journal of Sports Medicine*, researchers in

Switzerland noted that L-carnitine was in wide use by athletes as a dietary supplement, and reviewed literature available up to that time to see if such use was merited. They concluded that L-carnitine protects the heart and enhances its ability to tolerate stress; that although the evidence about the supplement's ability to enhance performance was somewhat contradictory, L-carnitine could be advantageous in sports. They noted that the supplement does improve aerobic capacity and can delay the formation of lactic acid in muscles, possibly extending endurance.

- In a study published in 1996 in a technical volume, *Carnitine–Pathobiochemical Basics and Clinical Applications,* German researchers examined what happens to carnitine during various types of intense exercise. They observed eleven well-trained male athletes who performed different types of exercise, and measured carnitine loss by testing urine and sweat. The researchers found that moderate exercise did not accelerate loss of carnitine, but extended or intense exercise did result in a greater loss of the nutrient. They observed that while significant amounts of carnitine were not lost in sweat as a result of exercise, carnitine loss through the urine was significantly greater in proportion to the quantity of extra calories being burned. The results suggested that people who engage in intense or extended exercise can benefit from L-carnitine supplementation.

- The results of research at the University of Connecticut at Storrs were published in two separate articles: one in the *Journal of Strength and Conditioning Research* in 2003, and another in *American Journal of Physiology Endocrinology and Metabolism* in 2002. In the trial, researchers examined the effect of L-carnitine on ten recreationally trained weight lifters. In this double-blind, placebo-controlled, crossover study, subjects were given 2 grams daily of the L-tartrate form of L-carnitine or a placebo for three weeks, and then performed five sets of fifteen to twenty repetitions of squat resistance exercises. After a one-week washout period to clear the subject's systems, those who had taken the placebo received L-carnitine and vice versa, and the exercises and tests were repeated. One of the tests after exercise, MRI scans of the mid-thigh area, showed 41 to 45 percent less tissue disruption when participants took L-carnitine before exercising during the three-week study period. In addition, L-carnitine resulted in significantly less free-radical generation caused by exercise. Participants also reported less soreness after taking L-carnitine during the four days following workout sessions.

- In 2004, researchers in Austria reviewed all the available research literature regarding the potential benefits of L-carnitine for athletes in an article published in the journal *Nutrition*. They concluded that L-carnitine may reduce muscle damage, promote recovery after exercise, and reduce levels of lactic acid that cause soreness, and offered potential benefit in training and competition.

Finding the Path to Results

The ideal exercise program generally includes three or more aerobic exercise workouts and two or three weight-training sessions per week. The idea is that a well-balanced program involves all of the parts of the body, including the heart and all the major muscle groups, to keep muscles strong and toned, and to counteract the loss of muscle mass that occurs as we age.

Some people cringe at the thought of going to

a health club and exercising in public. However, it's important to keep in mind that most of today's health clubs cater to a variety of age groups and fitness levels. Many offer exercise classes designed not only for beginners but also for people with limitations. These include classes such as water aerobics, to avoid stress on joints for those with osteoarthritis.

Health clubs do offer some advantages such as trained fitness professionals, who can show you how to perform movements to get maximum benefit without injury or too much stress on joints or muscles. They provide a variety of equipment and fitness classes to meet everyone's needs or preferences. And, most memberships include one or more one-on-one sessions with a trainer at no extra cost, which can be sufficient to get started on an appropriate and effective program.

However, you don't have to go to a gym to get regular exercise. Home workout videos or DVDs offer an endless variety of workouts for all fitness levels, from walking programs to yoga, complex dance moves, and an assortment of weight-training programs, or a combination of several approaches. While many of these require some type of equipment, it is usually inexpensive, such as light weights or stretchy bands that can be purchased for a few dollars at most sporting goods stores.

Another approach to fitness is to find activities you enjoy doing, like swimming, walking, playing tennis, golf (without the golf cart), or ballroom dancing. Social activities that include getting exercise are an enjoyable way to spend time with friends or get to know new people and keep exercise from being a chore.

Getting Started with an Exercise Program

Some of the most effective exercise strategies boil down to simple steps that can be incorporated

Providing Energy for Exercise

into most schedules. If you don't currently allocate time for exercise, try some of these approaches to get started:

- Set a realistic goal for a short period of time, such as a week, or even a day. For example, aim to go for a walk for twenty minutes during your lunch hour and for ten minutes during your coffee break. Write these down on your daily to-do list and check them off when they're done.

- Turn those walks into a daily habit, just like brushing your teeth.

- If you can't find a twenty-minute slot in your schedule, find a ten-minute one and aim to work in three ten-minute walks or other types of short exercise breaks during your day. Start by doing whatever you can and build from there.

- Set aside some time to explore health clubs. Many offer a free or very low-cost membership for a week or two. Try out a few different clubs before making a decision to purchase a membership.

- Turn some couch time into movement. When you watch television, get up and walk, jog in place, or do other exercises during commercials. Unless you're watching a commercial-free cable channel, you could get fifteen minutes of exercise during an hour-long program.

- Online, go to your favorite search engine and punch in "exercise videos." Read some reviews to get a sense of how different videos compare. To try videos without buying, you can borrow them from your local library, rent them from wherever you rent movies, or check your local TV listings for shows featuring exercise routines.

- If you have friends or coworkers who regularly go to an exercise or yoga class or to a nearby gym, ask them what they like about that particular workout. Consider trying it yourself.

Needless to say, it does require some will and a little planning to find the best way to get or stay in shape. L-carnitine can be a very helpful ingredient in a fitness strategy by helping your body produce energy more effectively. It will reduce the likelihood of "I'm too tired" being your excuse for staying inactive, missing opportunities to work out at the gym, or not getting involved in activities with friends.

A New Form of L-Carnitine

Richard Bloomer, Ph.D., director of the Cardiorespiratory/Metabolic Laboratory at the University of Memphis in Tennessee, has done an extensive amount of research in the area of exercise, oxidative stress, and nutrition, and is currently spearheading a study on the role of L-carnitine in exercise. After examining all the available research, he notes that the form of carnitine known as propionyl-L-carnitine has shown the greatest promise in relation to exercise benefits.

This form of carnitine was not available in the United States as a dietary supplement until recently, when AminoCarnitines were introduced by Sigma-tau HealthScience. This company has been producing L-carnitine for approximately thirty years, and has sponsored over 1,000 clinical trials with the nutrient. This type of L-carnitine supplement is based on science that shows that amino acids such as glycine, arginine, and lysine are related to L-carnitine's metabolic performance.

> **Amino Acids**
> *The components that make up proteins, vital parts of every cell in the human body.*

An AminoCarnitine is a molecule that contains both L-carnitine and an amino acid. The two substances are bound together until they reach the intestinal tract, where they break apart and are synergistically utilized by the body. Because the amino acid is bound with the L-carnitine in one molecule through a manufacturing process, the amounts of each substance and the quality of the formulation can be strictly controlled and standardized.

In his laboratory at the University of Memphis, Bloomer is studying the effect on exercise of an AminoCarnitine called glycine propionyl-L-carnitine hydrochloride, abbreviated GPLC. This product is available as AminoCarnitine and under the proprietary name of Ester Carnitine.

Propionyl-L-Carnitine and Exercise

"Propionyl-L-carnitine (PLC) is one of the most thoroughly researched forms of L-carnitine and may influence oxygen utilization, enhance athletic performance and improve health," says Bloomer. He explains that PLC, the propionyl form of L-carnitine in the AminoCarnitine dietary supplement, can reduce the degree of physical deterioration after a heart attack, a coronary artery bypass, or an angioplasty. "It has also been shown, in terms of blood lipid profile, to favorably alter the lipids," he says, "in general a decrease in total and the so-called bad cholesterol, the LDL, and the triglycerides, as well as an increase in good cholesterol, the HDL."

Lipids
Fats, including cholesterol and triglycerides, which are stored in the blood and body tissues and used for energy.

Earlier studies have found that levels of carnitine in muscles decrease when intense exercise is performed, and that process could be related to fatigue. Taking L-carnitine orally has been shown to replenish levels of carnitine in muscles, although the supplement usually needs to be taken for a month or more to significantly increase the amount of carnitine in skeletal muscle.

Bloomer's analysis of earlier L-carnitine research, combined with his personal research and work with athletes and patients, helps to explain how

User's Guide to L-Carnitine and Acetyl-L-Carnitine

GPLC can work in the body to enhance exercise performance. This is how it appears to work:

- It may increase carnitine content in the cells of the endothelium, the inner wall of blood vessels. This improves the blood vessels' ability to dilate and allows the muscle tissue to get more oxygen.

- It may increase circulation, which enables the heart to utilize more oxygen and get rid of toxic waste products more efficiently.

- The improved circulation and oxygen utilization may improve athletic performance.

- It may reduce the amount of oxidation caused by free radicals produced as a byproduct of exercise.

- By enhancing the utilization of fatty acids, energy in the form of ATP is produced more effectively and muscles use less glycogen (the carbohydrate stores in skeletal muscles).

- When carbohydrate, in the form of glycogen, is burned for energy, carnitine effectively removes waste products, resulting in more energy being generated from the glycogen. Carnitine facilitates less lactic acid production during high-intensity exercise by removing waste products as it does. Because lactic acid causes both pain and fatigue, fatigue and pain do not set in as quickly and endurance may be improved when less of it is produced.

> **Oxidation**
> *The process in which molecules are split by the addition of oxygen, resulting in free radicals, those compounds with an unpaired electron.*

- In high-intensity weight lifting, the supplement may reduce the inflammation and microtrauma to muscles that causes delayed-onset muscle soreness in the days following a workout.

Providing Energy for Exercise

In a nutshell, L-carnitine, particularly in the GPLC or Ester Carnitine form, enables your body to use more fatty acids during an intense workout, resulting in more efficient energy production and waste removal. The net effect is less lactic acid production, less pain and fatigue, and less damage by free radicals and inflammation to the heart and muscles.

"In other words, rather than failing after 120 minutes, a person potentially can go 130 minutes," says Bloomer. "While that may not seem like a lot for athletes or individuals involved in regular exercise, that's very, very important."

CHAPTER 4

ENHANCING WEIGHT LOSS

If you randomly select ten nutritional experts and ask them whether you should take L-carnitine to lose weight, chances are their responses will vary from a resounding "yes!" or "no!" to everywhere in between. However, if you ask physicians and nutritionists who specialize in weight loss, have a successful track record, and include dietary supplements in their regimens, L-carnitine is quite likely to be included in their program.

As an example, Certified Clinical Nutritionist Carol Simontacchi has been counseling people with weight problems for years, and has never advocated or condoned a quick-fix approach. She believes in a holistic strategy that includes education and results in permanent life changes and healthy weight. Her perspective on L-carnitine is simple: "Without sufficient L-carnitine, fats cannot be burned and instead will remain in the body." Simontacchi recommends taking 1 to 2 grams of L-carnitine per day, just before breakfast, as part of her comprehensive weight-loss program. This program is covered in detail in *Weight Success for a Lifetime* (Basic Health, 2005).

L-carnitine as a weight-loss aid is a topic on which experts frequently disagree, sometimes vehemently, as they do on other different diet strategies. For example, the Physician's Committee for Responsible Medicine (PCRM) is a Washington, D.C.-based, non-profit group that passionately promotes a vegetarian lifestyle, which does not include dairy products. As their name implies, the group's members include respected medical doctors, but people with credentials of similar stature do not necessarily agree with them when it comes to the conclusions of scientific investigations.

During the past few years, numerous research papers have been published in respected medical journals about the health benefits of dairy products, including data showing that dairy foods can promote weight loss. The dairy studies were also carried out by members of the medical profession who are not affiliated with PCRM. These two schools of thought—pro-dairy and anti-dairy—clash vehemently. While both sides seem to be supported by valid science that is accepted by the medical and academic communities, there seems to be no common ground.

> **Calorie**
> A unit of energy stored in the body through the consumption of food or drink or used as a result of living and activity.

When a leading food manufacturer launched a major advertising campaign promoting its dairy products as good foods to include in a weight-loss program, the PCRM took legal action to stop the campaign on the basis that the advertising was deceptive. The vegetarian group won in court and the food manufacturer withdrew its advertising campaign.

So, perhaps it's not surprising that there are varied perspectives about the benefits of L-carnitine for weight loss. However, contradictory medical opinions about weight loss run much deeper than this single disagreement.

Is Weight Loss Possible?

A few years ago, I moderated a panel of medical experts on weight loss at a conference. The difference of opinion among two comparably credentialed physicians on the panel was particularly dramatic. Both were board certified in bariatrics, the branch of medicine that specializes in treating obesity. Both were of similar age and had practiced medicine for a good twenty years. Both had invested exceptional amounts of time and effort to stay abreast of the latest science on the subject, and both had struggled with their own weight. However, their perspectives on the subject could not have been farther apart.

One expert focused on the theme that obesity is a complex, unfathomable problem without a foreseeable resolution, subtly conveying the message that anyone who claimed to have a solution to obesity was oversimplifying the issue. The key direction of action, according to this physician, should be to fund more research to gain a better understanding of the condition.

The other expert was equally confident, but had a perspective that was 180 degrees removed from the other physician: anyone could lose weight, given the right guidance and a sustainable strategy that would achieve optimum health, as well as a healthy weight, for the long term. On a personal level, this expert had successfully won the battle against obesity and was a picture of good health. In contrast, the other physician, who viewed obesity as an incurable disease, was visibly obese.

Could the difference in these two doctors' perspectives be attributed, at least partially, to their personal experiences? If someone succeeds at overcoming a physical condition, isn't it natural for him or her to believe that others can do the same? Even though human beings may be identically trained in medical science, perhaps their own experiences influence personal conviction more than scientific literature. On the other hand, perhaps the belief that one's physical condition can change makes it more likely that the pounds will come off.

Enhancing Weight Loss

Beliefs Matter in Results

Research does shed some light on how an individual's outlook influences their odds of success when trying to lose weight. A study published in the *Journal of the American Dietetic Association* found that you're more likely to lose weight if you believe you can control your eating habits and that excess weight is the consequence of your behavior and not from a physical origin, as compared to people who think their weight is beyond their control.

In this study, researchers in Holland established the beliefs of participants, forty-eight women and eighteen men with a body mass index (BMI) between thirty and fifty, by having them complete detailed questionnaires. The program consisted of an eight-week low-calorie diet supervised by a dietitian at an outpatient clinic. After comparing individual results of the program and individual beliefs, researchers concluded: "Although the low-calorie diet with meal replacements had a favorable effect on weight loss of all obese participants, individual differences in weight loss were predicted by beliefs at baseline." In other words, the success of each participant's outcome could have been predicted at the beginning of the study by looking at their completed questionnaire.

> **Body Mass Index (BMI)**
> *A measurement of body weight relative to height, used to determine whether a person is in a healthy, overweight, or obese range.*

The researchers also noted: "Eating behavior self-efficacy, the belief that one is able to regulate eating behavior, has been related to weight loss, eating habits, dietary behavior, and dietary self-care. Our study supports the idea that self-efficacy is a determinant of weight loss." In other words, if you believe that you can control your eating behavior, you're more likely to do so, and you will lose more weight as a result.

In the realm of beliefs, unrealistic goals are another common stumbling block. All too often, people set their goals at huge amounts of weight loss because of the common misconception that smaller amounts of weight loss are unimportant. However, if you're overweight, you will improve your health by losing between 7 and 10 percent of your body weight. Those are the findings of researchers at Baylor College of Medicine in Houston, Texas, in a study published in *Current Atherosclerosis Reports*. Even this level of weight loss can significantly reduce blood pressure, blood sugar, LDL ("bad") cholesterol, and triglycerides. The key lies in maintaining the loss.

Satisfying Your Appetite

Hunger drives people to eat, but L-carnitine lowers the risk of overeating by helping your body utilize food more efficiently for energy. There is a visible correlation, although the mechanism isn't fully understood by scientists. Swiss researchers who reviewed all the scientific literature on the subject and published their findings in *Physiology and Behavior* noted: "Fatty acid oxidation is thought to play a role in the control of food intake."

Earlier animal research has shown that rats automatically eat more when their ability to turn fats into energy is diminished. In contrast, when rats are given substances known to increase the burning of fats for energy, they eat less. Carnitine enhances the body's ability to turn fats into energy, and also helps support the function of insulin in utilizing sugars as energy.

Foods That Satisfy

There is plenty of clinical experience and numerous studies demonstrating that certain types of food are more satisfying than others when it comes to satisfying the human appetite. A food does not have to be high in calories to be satisfy-

Enhancing Weight Loss

ing. In fact, some low-calorie foods can be much more satisfying than rich, sugary ones, although the latter are often the first choice when hunger pangs strike.

Water-rich foods, including all types of vegetables and fruits, are rich in antioxidants and many other nutrients and can be eaten in almost unlimited amounts, as long as they aren't doctored with high-calorie, nutrient-poor sauces, garnishes, or condiments. For example, virtually all types of raw vegetables that can be included in salads are high in water and nutrients known to prevent every imaginable disease, including cancer, diabetes, and heart disease. They are naturally low in calories unless they're covered in unhealthy, high-fat dressings. Even potatoes can be a healthy food if they're baked and eaten with salsa instead of being fried or eaten with liberal amounts of butter, sour cream, bacon bits, or other high-fat, high-calorie, nutrient-poor toppings. These same healthy foods are high in fiber, a component that is literally a no-calorie ingredient, because it acts like a freight train traveling through our system and taking some unhealthy calories with it. Fats and sugars are absorbed to a lesser degree when a diet contains a healthy dose of fiber, which is also a food that is high on the satisfaction scale.

Eating a higher proportion of protein also makes a significant impact on appetite, according to a study at the University of Washington School of Medicine in Seattle. In a study published in the *American Journal of Clinical Nutrition,* researchers tested different ratios of protein, fat, and carbohydrates on nineteen people and found that eating more protein curbs appetite and results in fewer total calories being eaten, even when there is no conscious restriction of calories.

Based on the above, good and satisfying dietary choices include baked or boiled potatoes, popcorn (go very easy on the butter), high-fiber cereals such as oatmeal, apples, oranges, grapes, whole-grain pasta, lentils, beans, eggs, very lean beef such as top round, and fish that isn't fatty, such as cod.

During a twelve-week diet containing 30 percent protein, 20 percent fat, and 50 percent carbohydrate, nineteen overweight study participants—who could eat all they wanted as long as they maintained the 30-20-50 ratio—spontaneously ate 441 calories less per day than they had been eating previously, and lost an average of eleven pounds. An important point of this type of diet is to eat healthy carbohydrates, fresh vegetables, and whole grains, rather than processed foods. And, for optimum health, the protein sources should be lean.

Carbohydrates, Good and Bad

There is a lot of confusion when it comes to carbohydrates. It's helpful to get a little understanding about how different types of carbohydrates work in your body, so that you can make informed choices for achieving or maintaining a healthy weight. L-carnitine is a key tool for losing excess fat, but it's important to look at the bigger picture of weight loss before we get to that, because there is no substitute for a healthy lifestyle. Once that's in place, L-carnitine and other supplements can truly help you to achieve an optimum weight and state of health.

One of the reasons carbohydrates became somewhat unpopular in recent years is because some of them convert very rapidly to blood sugar. This causes rapid spikes in energy, followed by rapid slumps that lead to cravings and overeating. The body has to produce insulin to shuttle the blood sugar, or glucose, from blood to tissues to be used as energy. However, the whole insulin mechanism has started to malfunction in many people, because the American diet has become so rich in refined and sugary foods. The most com-

Enhancing Weight Loss

mon result of our unhealthy diet is a condition known as Syndrome X or prediabetes, where insulin is unable to get the glucose into tissue and the energy is stored as fat instead.

It's a vicious cycle where the body can't use energy properly, and keeps shuttling more fuel to fat instead of burning it. Controlling the type and quantity of carbohydrates that are eaten can start reversing the cycle, and that's where "low-glycemic" diets enter the picture.

Glucose
A simple sugar that is the main source of energy for cellular and bodily functions.

"Glycemic" literally means that there is glucose in the blood. Foods that convert to glucose slowly are categorized as "low-glycemic" foods and those that convert quickly are "high-glycemic." There is a glycemic index (GI) that rates dozens of foods from highest ranking (highest glycemic-index) foods to lowest, which has given rise to a new diet buzzword: low-GI. Before being included in the index, each food was tested in a lab to see how quickly it converts to blood sugar when compared to other foods and to pure glucose.

Glycemic Index
A ranking of foods based on how much they cause blood sugar to rise in a specific period of time.

The glycemic index was originally developed for research purposes, rather than for your dinner table. Consequently, when it rates foods, it does not take into account how much of a given food you're likely to eat. For example, carrots rate higher than white bread on the index, yet carrots are healthy vegetables which react quite differently in your system than white bread. You would have to eat approximately one and a half pounds of carrots to generate the same amount of blood sugar from carrots as you would from one slice of the bread. People just don't eat like that, even in eating contests.

Another way to measure the impact of a food

on your blood sugar is called the glycemic load. This is how a food's glycemic load is calculated: The amount of carbohydrate in a food is established, and its impact on blood sugar is calculated based on that quantity. For example, the carbohydrate in carrots converts rapidly into blood sugar. However, only 4 percent of a carrot is carbohydrate. So even though the carbohydrate in carrots rapidly turns to blood sugar, it doesn't have a big impact because it is such a small amount. Bottom line: Carrots are good for you.

As a rule of thumb, if you eat foods that are pretty close to their natural state instead of processed foods, you will be eating foods that do not cause problems with blood sugar because they are low in glycemic load. For most people, this is easier said than done. For example, few people today routinely eat real vegetables on a day-to-day basis, whether raw, steamed, or lightly grilled. (For a list of foods that have a low-glycemic load, see Appendix B.)

> **Low-Glycemic**
> Foods that convert to blood sugar slowly, eliminating blood-sugar spikes.

Other Appetite Control Strategies

Skipping breakfast can make you eat more during the course of a day. British researchers came to this conclusion after monitoring ten lean women's total daily food intake when they did and didn't eat breakfast. In the study, also published in the *American Journal of Clinical Nutrition*, the women ate a breakfast of bran cereal with low-fat milk for two weeks, then no breakfast for another two weeks. During both time periods, they ate two snacks and two meals later in the day. Researchers found that not only did the women eat more on no-breakfast days, but their cholesterol levels were higher and their bodies' sensitivity to insulin decreased, indicating that their ability to utilize blood sugar was diminished.

Enhancing Weight Loss

Sleep also influences appetite and the probability of weight gain. "Sleeping less could serve as a trigger to the body to increase food intake and store fat," said lead researcher James Gangwisch, Ph.D., at Columbia University in New York City. His research, presented at a scientific meeting of the North American Association for the Study of Obesity, found that people who slept four hours or less per night were 73 percent more likely to be obese than those who slept between seven and nine hours. Five hours of sleep increased risk of obesity by 50 percent; and six hours of shut eye raised risk by 23 percent.

"The results are somewhat counterintuitive, since people who sleep less are naturally burning more calories," said Gangwisch. "But we think it has more to do with what happens to your body when you deprive it of sleep as opposed to the amount of physical activity that you get."

Sleep deprivation seems to trick appetite-regulating hormones into thinking you need more food than you actually do. Gangwisch thinks our ancestors' lifestyles could help to explain why this happens: "The metabolic regulatory system may have evolved to motivate humans to store fat during summer months when the nights are shorter and food is plentiful, which was a survival mechanism for the body to prepare for the dark winter months when food would not be as plentiful. As a result, sleeping less could serve as a trigger to the body to increase food intake and store fat."

In another study, researchers at East Virginia Medical School in Norfolk, Virginia, examined the sleeping habits of 1,001 people and compared sleep times with body mass index (BMI). In the study, published in the *Archives of Internal Medicine*, they concluded that as little as twenty minutes of extra sleep per night correlates with a lower BMI. According to the study, the more you sleep, the less likely you are to be overweight, although the premise doesn't hold true for extremely obese people.

Weight-Loss Basics

People who have lost weight and keep it off inevitably follow certain basic principles. The National Weight Control Registry is a database created by obesity experts from several leading universities in the United States to track how people effectively achieve and maintain a healthy weight. The database includes approximately 4,000 people who have lost at least thirty pounds and kept it off for at least a year, and the basic message boils down to this:

- Lasting weight loss requires permanent changes in diet.

- People who successfully reduce their weight and keep it off pay attention to the types of foods they eat and how much they eat. They moderate their intake of fat and total calories.

- Successful weight losers exercise, often for an hour per day on most days of the week, and usually do some type of moderate exercise, such as walking.

- Nearly half of those who have lost and kept weight off for some years say that it's easier to maintain their new, healthy weight than it was to lose the pounds.

Once your healthy diet and exercise program is established, adding the right supplements can improve results and ensure that your body is getting nutrients that support your best intentions and efforts. L-carnitine is a key nutrient to support weight loss and maintenance.

L-Carnitine: The "Fat Burner"

When people talk about dietary supplements that

Enhancing Weight Loss

are "fat burners," they are usually referring to substances that speed up the body's metabolism. Ephedra became well known for this before it was banned as a potential health risk, although the degree of danger it posed still remains a controversial issue. Caffeine has a similar effect. The net effect of stimulants is that your body is tricked into believing that you're walking faster than you really are, or moving a bit when you're really sitting still. And, one of the side effects of any stimulant can be an uncomfortable jittery or nervous feeling.

L-carnitine doesn't work in this fashion but it does, literally, enhance the burning of fat. Rather than tricking your metabolism into functioning at an artificially altered, higher rate like caffeine and ephedra, L-carnitine enables mitochondria in cells to convert fats from the food you eat into energy molecules known as ATP. Your body uses the ATP as the fuel for everything it does to stay alive and perform whatever level of exertion you choose. One could say that L-carnitine's fat-burning action occurs at a much more basic level than that of a stimulant.

How might L-carnitine's fat-burning attribute manifest itself in terms of how it makes you feel? You may not notice any obvious difference, because there isn't any "rush" type of effect. However, you may notice that you have the energy to do more things than you used to, or that you no longer feel the need to reach for a snack as a pick-me-up at times when you aren't hungry. Or, if you've experienced feeling more tired than usual a day or two after some type of exercise, you may find that this is no longer the case.

Research Findings

There is no dispute among scientists about the role of the carnitine molecule in human metabolism. They agree that it is necessary for fats to be converted to energy. And, numerous studies have demonstrated that L-carnitine enhances the ability of our cells to perform that function when it is used as dietary supplement.

For example, one recent study carried out in Germany and published in the journal *Metabolism* analyzed breath and urine samples of twelve people on a weight-loss diet. Researchers tracked how fat and protein were utilized with and without supplementation. They found that L-carnitine (subjects took 1.5 grams of the L-tartrate form three times daily) significantly increased the conversion of fat to energy.

In contrast, studies that have measured the amount of weight lost with and without an L-carnitine supplement have had mixed results, although some have demonstrated a clear weight-loss benefit. One possible explanation for differing outcomes is that some studies did not last long enough to effectively measure the impact of the nutrient. Or, differences in testing protocols may influence the variation in findings.

An Enlightening Study

Among the various studies of L-carnitine's role in weight loss, there is one that was carried out with an unusual level of precision in measuring changes in body fat. Its findings shed some light on how and why the supplement belongs in weight-loss programs. This study was a joint effort between researchers at the University of Texas in San Antonio and Harbor-UCLA Medical Center in Torrance, California, and was published in *Current Therapeutic Research* in 1992.

In the study, thirty obese women and ten obese men between the ages of nineteen and sixty-eight did two eight-week programs, the first without any supplements and the second with L-carnitine, the mineral chromium, and high-fiber cookies designed to be used in a weight-loss plan. In both phases, the participants ate a low-calorie diet, consisting of an average of 1,249 daily calories for women and 1,653 daily calories for men.

A major problem with low-calorie diets is that as people lose weight, their resting metabolic rate (RMR), measured by the calories required for all the basic processes of life, decreases. A lower RMR increases the risk of weight gain and is one of the key reasons why people regain weight. In addition, low-calorie diets can also lead to reduced lean body mass, which in turn reduces strength as well as RMR and also promotes weight gain. These were major issues that this trial was designed to address.

One of the unusual aspects of this study was the method used to measure body fat. Usually researchers rely on calipers to measure fat in various parts of the body or on electrical impedance. In the latter, a person lies down with electrodes attached, similar to the electrodes used in echocardiograms but positioned in different parts of the body. A tiny, imperceptible current runs through the body and the percentage of body fat is calculated on the basis of electrical resistance since lean mass provides greater resistance than fat mass. Neither of these two methods is considered to be the most accurate measure of body fat, but they are economical and relatively convenient to do.

One of the most accurate ways to determine body fat is underwater weighing, in which an individual is literally submerged in water. The method is based on the premise that fat is less dense than lean body mass. During the test, a person is weighed out of the water and in the water, and density, including lean mass and fat mass, is calculated using mathematical formulas. Despite its relatively greater accuracy, this method is not used as often as the others because it is much more cumbersome and requires a special testing laboratory.

In this weight-loss study, researchers used the

underwater weighing method to measure body fat and lean mass at the outset and at various stages of the trial. They found that during the first eight weeks, there was no significant change in body composition or cholesterol levels when participants were given individual diets designed to be appropriate for their individual RMR and followed an exercise program.

During the second eight weeks, the loss of body fat averaged approximately one and a half pounds per week when supplements of L-carnitine, chromium, and fiber were added. At the same time, their lean body mass was preserved and their metabolism improved, with RMR increasing from an average of 1,126 to 1,367. In other words, the basic daily caloric requirements required by these people while at rest increased by an average of 240 calories daily, or 21 percent. Such an increase is very significant as it overcomes one of the stumbling blocks of weight maintenance—the fact that typically, people need fewer calories per day as they lose weight, making weight regain difficult to avoid.

Researchers also noted that participants found it easier to adhere to their diet during the second phase, when they were taking supplements. In addition, the supplements had a positive effect on cholesterol levels: during the first phase of the trial, there were no changes in cholesterol, but during the supplement phase, total and LDL ("bad") cholesterol levels significantly decreased.

Other Research

L-carnitine has been studied as an aid to weight loss for some time. In 1986, one researcher wrote in the journal *Medical Hypotheses*, "The efficacy of low-fat diets may be promoted by supplementary carnitine, which stimulates fat oxidation, and by chromium, which aids insulin-mediated thermogenesis. An unrefined low-fat diet, eaten to satiety and accompanied by regular exercise, may be the ideal means of maintaining a trim figure throughout life while minimizing one's risk for 'Western' degenerative diseases."

In research published in 1998 in a German scientific journal *Medical Journal for Natural Therapy*, L-carnitine's effect was tested on 100 obese people, in conjunction with a diet and moderate exercise. The participants were divided into two groups, both following a 1,200-calorie diet, but one group also took L-carnitine supplements. The supplement group lost 25 percent more weight than the other group.

The researchers noted that in calorie-restricted diets that limit fat, people often eat less red meat, the key dietary source of carnitine. Therefore, there may be a deficiency of L-carnitine in such diets, and supplements may be especially helpful to ensure that energy is generated efficiently from the fat that is in the diet.

Scientists have also identified a connection between L-carnitine and efficient insulin function, which is often compromised in people who are obese or overweight. For example, in 2003, a study published in *Acta Diabetologica* noted, "The carnitine system is shown to be determinant in insulin regulation of fat and glucose metabolic rate in skeletal muscle, this being critical in determining body composition and relevant raised levels of risk factors for cardiovascular disease, obesity, hypertension, and type 2 diabetes."

CHAPTER 5

ACETYL-L-CARNITINE, AGING, AND MENTAL DECLINE

In 2002, a group of rats in Northern California grabbed media attention around the world. "These old rats got up and did the Macarena," was one of the most quoted statements about the animals, who were not in a circus but in a research laboratory.

The statement came from Bruce Ames, Ph.D., lead researcher in a series of studies that broke new ground in the subject of aging. Ames and his colleagues at the University of California, Berkeley and the Children's Hospital Oakland Research Institute discovered that a combination of two nutritional supplements—acetyl-L-carnitine, a specific form of L-carnitine, and alpha-lipoic acid—enabled old rats to function like their much younger peers.

Tory Hagan, Ph.D., who worked on the research with Ames, summed up their findings this way: "We significantly reversed the decline in overall activity typical of aged rats to what you see in a middle-aged to young adult rat seven to 10 months of age. This is equivalent to making a 75 to 80-year-old person act middle-aged."

The research found that after a month of supplements, previously old, lethargic rats functioned in a much younger way, both physically and mentally. In addition to a rebound in energy levels, their memories, measured with mentally challenging tests, were like those of young animals, as was their appearance. Examination of various tissues showed that mitochondria showed significantly less decay in the supplemented rats' brain cells than those in brain cells of rats not fed the supplements. In essence, the supplements were able to protect and rejuvenate the mitochondria in the animals' cells.

More recently, Hagan stated in the *Journal of the American Medical Association:* "Experiments that caused mice to quickly develop characteristics of premature aging reveal that mutations in mitochondrial DNA may play a key role in growing old." She summed up the new research this way: "For years, mitochondria have been linked to aging. In the new findings, researchers demonstrated that an accumulation of genetic mutations in mitochondria sets off a cascade of signals that causes programmed cell death, or apoptosis. The result is loss of irreplaceable cells and progression of aging."

> **DNA**
> Deoxyribonucleic acid, the molecule that carries genetic information in all living organisms.

Acetyl-L-Carnitine (ALC)

The ALC form of L-carnitine is particularly well utilized by the brain and nervous system because it crosses the blood-brain barrier. Bruce Ames is one of numerous researchers who have established this fact. In 2004, he presented later research to an international conference, *Carnitine: The Science Behind a Conditionally Essential Nutrient*, sponsored by several of the entities that comprise the United States government's National Institutes of Health and Office of Dietary Supplements.

At the conference, Ames presented findings from one of his clinical trials with rats to compare the effects of acetyl-L-carnitine and L-carnitine supplements. His research showed that both types of carnitine supplements were effective at improving the rats' energy levels and ability to move. However, the ALC supplements were significantly more effective at preserving mitochondria in brain cells, and acted as an antioxidant for brain tissues. This helps to explain why ALC is particularly effective in enhancing the function of memory and disorders related to the central nervous system, such as diabetic neuropathy, which will be discussed in the next chapter. ALC has also improved age-related hearing loss in animal research.

Ames also presented a comprehensive review of research regarding ALC. In his review, he stated: "A recent meta-analysis of twenty-one double-blind clinical trials of ALC in the treatment of mild cognitive impairment and mild AD [Alzheimer's disease] showed significant efficacy vs. placebo." That review examined studies in which participants took a form of ALC known as ALCAR, in amounts ranging from 1.5 to 3 grams daily, for at least three months. Clinical and psychometric tests demonstrated benefits after three months of supplementation, and the positive effects of ALCAR increased over time. The supplement was well tolerated by the study participants.

Aging and Disease

The theory that deterioration in mitochondria accelerates aging and age-related disabilities is gaining more prominence in scientific circles. Certainly, the condition of mitochondria influences many disease states. "If you can delay the onset of the mitochondria becoming ill, or becoming dysfunctional, you can delay the onset of disease," says Stephen Sinatra, M.D. In addition to decreased ability to exercise, lower energy levels, and heart disease, other conditions connected with deteriorating mitochondria include prediabetes (also called Syndrome X), diabetes, diabetic neuropathy, memory loss, Alzheimer's disease, Parkinson's disease, multiple sclerosis, arthritis, cancer, chronic fatigue syndrome, fibromyalgia, male infertility, aging of the skin, age-related macular degeneration, and hearing loss.

Acetyl-L-Carnitine, Aging, and Mental Decline

The relationship of L-carnitine to some of these conditions has been covered in earlier chapters, and its relationship to diabetes and male infertility are covered in the following chapters. This is some of the research relating to ALC and other conditions:

- A double-blind, placebo-controlled trial in Italy examined the impact of ALC, omega-3 fatty acids, and CoQ_{10} on age-related macular degeneration (AMD). In the study, published in *Ophthalmologica*, 106 people diagnosed with early AMD were given either a placebo or a combination of the three supplements. The supplement group showed significant improvement after twelve months.

- A study of thirty people with chronic fatigue syndrome, published in 2004 in *Psychosomatic Medicine*, found that both ALC and propionyl-L-carnitine (available as Ester Carnitine) improved fatigue and attention concentration.

- In 2004, a randomized, placebo-controlled, crossover study of thirty-six multiple sclerosis patients published in the *Journal of Neurological Sciences* found that 1 gram twice daily of ALC (ALCAR) was more effective at reducing fatigue and better tolerated than the medication amantadine.

- In 2004, ALC (ALCAR) was tested for up to thirty-three months on twenty-one patients suffering from peripheral neuropathy from *human immunodeficiency virus* (HIV) medications. In the open trial, published in *AIDS*, 1.5 grams twice daily of ALCAR improved symptoms and helped peripheral nerves to regenerate.

- In 2005, intravenous ALC was tested on twenty-seven cancer patients suffering from peripheral neuropathy as a side effect of treatment. In the pilot study, published in *Tumori—a Journal of*

Experimental and Clinical Oncology, 73 percent of the patients experienced significant relief after ALC treatment for ten to twenty days.

Warding off diseases that are more likely to develop with age is one way of staying young. Many people want more: they want the level of energy they had in earlier years. ALC combined with alpha-lipoic acid may help to accomplish both goals.

CHAPTER 6

L-CARNITINE, ACETYL-L-CARNITINE, DIABETES, AND PREDIABETES

There are more than 18 million people suffering from diabetes in the United States, according to the American Diabetes Association (ADA), although about 5 million of these don't even know they have the disease. The most common form of the disease is type 2 diabetes, often called non-insulin dependent diabetes, which typically develops later in life and is significantly influenced by unhealthy lifestyles. Its incidence is growing rapidly.

In addition, the ADA estimates that there are another 41 million Americans who have prediabetes, a condition that leads to diabetes. In prediabetes, insulin does not function properly. This causes blood sugar levels to be elevated, although not to the same extent as in the disease itself. L-carnitine may help with both prediabetes and diabetes.

One of the debilitating consequences of diabetes is nerve damage, or diabetic neuropathy. Whether it is type 1 diabetes, which usually begins in childhood, or type 2 diabetes, which usually begins in adulthood, it is estimated that about half of diabetics suffer some type of nerve damage. This is one area where acetyl-L-carnitine has been shown to bring about significant improvement.

Diabetic Neuropathy

A survey by the American Diabetes Association found that while most diabetics experience some degree of nerve damage as a result of their disease, only one in four have been diagnosed with this condition. More than half of those who experience symptoms don't know that the condition is called diabetic neuropathy.

There are two types of diabetic neuropathy: peripheral, which affects the hands and feet, and autonomic, which affects other parts of the body. Symptoms of peripheral neuropathy include tingling, pain, numbness, or weakness in your feet and hands. The feet may be so sensitive that wearing socks or touching bed sheets can cause pain. Numbness may make a person unaware of a foot injury. This type of nerve damage can lead to food ulcers, infections, and, in severe cases, amputation.

> **Diabetic Neuropathy**
> Nerve damage that is a complication of diabetes.

Symptoms of autonomic neuropathy can include digestive problems, nausea, vomiting, diarrhea, constipation, bladder problems, difficulty having sex, dizziness or feeling faint, increased or decreased sweating, changes in how the eyes react to light and dark, and an inability to perceive signs of low blood sugar or even typical signs of a heart attack. When nerve damage is in the early stages, it may be reversible, but as it progresses, structural changes become permanent.

Acetyl-L-Carnitine and Nerve Damage

Numerous studies have shown that acetyl-L-carnitine (ALC) is deficient in diabetics, and that the supplement can significantly help lessen the nerve damage caused by diabetes. In 2005, the journal *Diabetes Care* published the results of two large studies led by researchers at Wayne State University in Detroit, Michigan.

The two trials, which were double-blind and placebo-controlled, involved 1,257 patients in multiple treatment centers in the United States, Canada, and Europe. All of these patients had been diagnosed with diabetic neuropathy. During the trials, patients took either 500 milligrams or 1,000 milligrams of ALC or a placebo three times daily for one year. The higher dosage produced better results, and improvement was greater in type 2 diabetics who had suffered from the disease for the shortest period of time. Nerve damage is known to be less severe in type 2 diabetes than with type 1, and damage is progressive, so earlier treatment produces the greatest effect. Type 2 diabetics whose blood sugar was not well controlled experienced some of the most noticeable improvements.

Researchers performed microscopic examinations of nerve fibers, measured how quickly nerves transmit information, tested vibration perception, and analyzed other symptoms of diabetic neuropathy, including pain. They found that patients taking ALC were experiencing relief by the twenty-sixth week of the trial. During these trials, patients experienced significant pain relief and an improved ability to perceive vibration, and tests showed improvement in nerve structure and some regeneration of nerve fibers. Speed of nerve conduction did not change, however.

Preventing Diabetes

Scientific analysis of various systems in the body shows that carnitine is instrumental not only in burning fat for energy, but also in enabling insulin to do its job of shuttling glucose, or blood sugar, to cells so that it can be burned as fuel. This role of the nutrient offers a valuable benefit for diabetics, those at high risk for the disease, and also for healthy people.

Some studies have tested the direct effect of L-carnitine on glucose by testing people after intravenous L-carnitine infusions. For example, in a study published in 2000 in *Metabolism*, ALC was administered intravenously to eighteen type 2 diabetics and significantly improved their utilization of glucose. Earlier, similar research also found that the supplement also improves glucose utilization in type 1 diabetics and in healthy people.

In prediabetes, where glucose is elevated and the risk of diabetes is increased, insulin is not able to get glucose into cells because the cells do not respond—hence the term "insulin resistance." There are a number of lifestyle factors that contribute to this condition (see below). A diet with a good balance of protein, low-glycemic carbohydrates and healthy fats, regular exercise, and a healthy weight are all necessary for a diabetes-free life, but L-carnitine and other supplements also promote healthy insulin function and help prevent diabetes. Other useful supplements include alpha-lipoic acid, chromium, vanadyl sulfate, and omega-3 fatty acids.

> **Insulin**
> A hormone that transports glucose to tissues and enables the body to use it as fuel.

Lifestyle Factors That May Contribute to Insulin Resistance

- Weight gain
- Abdominal fat
- Lack of physical activity
- A diet lacking nutritious, lean protein
- Deficiency of healthy fats, especially omega-3 fatty acids found in fish
- Low vegetable intake
- Too many high-glycemic foods
- Too much refined sugar and flour
- Too little fiber

CHAPTER 7

IMPROVING MALE FERTILITY

One factor that makes conception difficult is reduced sperm motility, or an inability of sperm to swim as they need to so they can reach and fertilize an egg. A number of studies have shown that carnitine supplements may help in these cases.

One double-blind, placebo-controlled study, published in *Fertility and Sterility* in 2004, tracked fifty-six men between the ages of twenty and forty for six months. All of the participants had reduced sperm motility. Half the men took a placebo, while the other half took a combination of 2 grams of L-carnitine and 1 gram of acetyl-L-carnitine daily. Tests showed that sperm motility improved significantly among those taking the carnitine combination.

The health of mitochondria plays a role in the impact of L-carnitine in these cases, as it does in other conditions. One study, published in the same journal a year later, found that the effect of carnitine supplements on sperm motility is greater if mitochondria are healthier to begin with. Researchers studied thirty men, with an average age of thirty-four, who had experienced fertility problems and had reduced sperm motility. The men took a placebo for three months, then 2 grams of L-carnitine for another three months. Their sperm was tested before and after each regimen and three months after treatment ended.

Researchers found that sperm motility increased with carnitine, but it did so to a greater extent when mitochondrial function was normal at the outset, and to a lesser extent where mitochondria were compromised to some degree. The placebo produced no change. When semen was tested three months after supplements were stopped, some minor improvement was still evident, but sperm motility relapsed for the most part after carnitine supplementation ended.

L-carnitine supplements have also been shown to affect other aspects of sperm quality. A study of 170 infertile men, published in *Drugs R&D* in 2005, included men with and without decreased sperm motility. Participants received 1 gram of L-carnitine plus 1 gram of acetyl-L-carnitine daily. Tests after three and six months showed that carnitine content in semen correlated with sperm motility, sperm concentration, cellular integrity, sperm count, and overall sperm quality in all participants.

> **Sperm Motility**
> *The ability of sperm to move effectively and be able to fertilize an egg.*

Men and Aging

L-carnitine may be more effective and less risky than testosterone as a tool to slow the aging process in men. In a study of male aging published in 2004 in *Urology*, 120 men with a mean age of sixty-six were divided into three groups. One group was given testosterone, another was given a placebo, and the third was given a combination of 2 grams of ALC and 2 grams of propionyl-L-carnitine. Various parameters of aging were tracked, including age-related aspects of prostate health and sexual function, depression, and fatigue. None of the groups experienced improvements in prostate condition, but the size of the prostate increased after three months in the testosterone group. Once the testosterone was discontinued, the prostate size decreased within six months but did not return to its original size.

Improving Male Fertility

Sexual function and satisfaction improved in the testosterone and carnitine groups after three months, and improved further in the carnitine group after six months. Fatigue decreased and mood improved significantly in the same two groups, but more so in the carnitine group. And, the improvement in erectile function, orgasm, and sexual well-being was significantly greater after six months in the carnitine group. Overall, the carnitine supplements provided the greatest improvement in all respects, without any risk factors.

Peyronie's disease is a condition in which plaque forms a benign but painful lump on the penis and may cause a curvature. It occurs most often in middle-aged men. Several studies have shown that carnitine supplementation can help to alleviate this condition. One, published in *BJU International* in 2001, compared the effects of 1 gram twice daily of acetyl-L-carnitine and tamoxifen, a medication. Among forty-eight patients, which included both chronic sufferers and those who had recently developed the disease, ALC was significantly more effective than tamoxifen in reducing pain, inhibiting progression of the disease, and reducing curvature, without side effects. In contrast, tamoxifen induced significant side effects and did not reduce curvature.

CHAPTER 8

THE CARNITINE PROGRAM

The previous chapters have shown how L-carnitine can improve your health and ensure the quality of your life. These basic lifestyle habits will maximize the benefits of L-carnitine:

- Get at least thirty minutes of exercise daily on most days of the week. Include aerobic activity and two to three sessions of resistance training per week.

- Eat a healthy diet that supports a normal weight. Choose foods as close to their natural state as possible, rather than processed food products. Choose lean proteins, including at least two to three servings of cold-water fish (good sources of healthy omega-3 fats) per week, and include fresh vegetables, raw ones where possible, with each meal. For snacks, opt for fresh fruit or vegetables and/or raw nuts in moderation.

L-Carnitine Forms and Dosages

In addition to the following dosages and supplements, take a good-quality daily multivitamin/mineral supplement for overall nutritional support. If any of the nutrients in the following lists are also included in your multisupplement, include that amount when calculating your daily total.

For Heart Health, Exercise Support, and Weight Loss

- Take either L-carnitine or the AminoCarnitine GPLC (glycine propionyl-L-carnitine hydrochlo-

The Carnitine Program

ride), also known as Ester Carnitine, according to the following directions and dosages:

- GPLC or Ester Carnitine: 1.6 to 3.2 grams once or twice daily on an empty stomach, before breakfast or lunch. For athletes, take an additional 1.6 to 3.2 gram dose one hour before an intense workout.
- L-carnitine: 500 milligrams to 3 grams daily.

- CoQ_{10}: 90 to 260 milligrams daily.
- D-ribose: 5 to 15 grams daily. Serious athletes can take up to 20 grams daily.
- Magnesium: 400 to 800 milligrams daily.
- Fish oil: 1 to 3 grams daily.

For Healthy Aging and Brain Health

- Acetyl-L-carnitine: 500 milligrams acetyl-L-carnitine two to three times daily.
- Alpha-lipoic acid: 200 milligrams two to three times daily.

For Diabetes Prevention

- Acetyl-L-carnitine: 500 milligrams two to three times daily.
- Alpha-lipoic acid: 600 milligrams daily.
- Chromium: 250 to 500 micrograms twice daily.
- Vanadyl sulfate: 1 milligram daily.
- Fish oil: 1 to 3 grams daily.

For Male Fertility

- L-carnitine and acetyl-L-carnitine: 1 to 2 grams of each per day.
- ProXeed: This supplement is a combination of the two forms of carnitine designed for male fertility support, and is available at www.proxeed.com.

For Multiple Benefits

If your objective is to prevent multiple conditions, combine the supplements listed above for each condition. Where the same supplement is listed in more than one section, there is no need to duplicate doses. For example, if your objective is to prevent heart disease and diabetes, 1 to 3 grams of fish oil is sufficient.

Where different types of carnitine supplements are recommended, take each of the different types, as each one is particularly helpful for the stated conditions. For example, propionyl-L-carnitine in GPLC and Ester Carnitine is particularly beneficial for heart health, whereas acetyl-L-carnitine is particularly beneficial for aging, brain health, and diabetes. For optimum health in all these respects, take the recommended dosage of each type of carnitine.

Conclusion

The information in this User's Guide can be used in many ways. If you or someone you care about is suffering from a disease that L-carnitine or acetyl-L-carnitine could help treat, consult your physician about implementing the supplement in your treatment program. If the response is less than positive, keep in mind that medical opinions differ widely. Seek out a second or even a third opinion from a physician who is well versed in treating the condition and is familiar, or at least willing to investigate, a more comprehensive approach that utilizes one or both of these supplements.

If you care about your health and know that you are not in the best shape you could be, I encourage you to try L-carnitine, acetyl-L-carnitine, or the new AminoCarnitine, also known as Ester Carnitine. However, I also encourage you to use the supplement as just that—a supplement—rather than as a substitute for healthy lifestyle choices. The supplement can still help if your diet and exercise habits fall far short of ideal, but it's a little like constantly bailing water from a leaky boat instead of using the best possible tools to repair the boat and maintain its condition.

Our health is challenged in today's world by a lack of opportunities to exert ourselves physically and a lack of nutritious food choices. Harness L-carnitine's potential to the fullest, by using it along with food and exercise habits that foster good health. As a nutrient that enhances your body's production of energy at a basic cellular level, L-carnitine is a tool that can jumpstart your path to well-being.

APPENDIX A

BODY MASS INDEX

Health professionals use body mass index (BMI) to determine if a person is underweight, normal weight, overweight, or obese. Health risks are greater for overweight people and even greater still for those who are obese.

To find your BMI on the chart, find your height in the row on the left, then look across the chart to find your weight. Your BMI will be at the top of that column. The chart may not be accurate for a minority of people who are very lean but have unusually large amounts of muscle. For most people, this is what BMI numbers indicate:

- Underweight: BMI equal to or less than 18.5
- Normal weight: BMI is between 18.5 and 24.9
- Overweight: BMI is between 25 and 29.9
- Obesity: BMI is 30 or greater

BMI	19	20	21	22	23	24	25	26
Height (inches)				Body Weight (pounds)				
58	91	96	100	105	110	115	119	124
59	94	99	104	109	114	119	124	128
60	97	102	107	112	118	123	128	133
61	100	106	111	116	122	127	132	137
62	104	109	115	120	126	131	136	142
63	107	113	118	124	130	135	141	146
64	110	116	122	128	134	140	145	151
65	114	120	126	132	138	144	150	156
66	118	124	130	136	142	148	155	161
67	121	127	134	140	146	153	159	166
68	125	131	138	144	151	158	164	171
69	128	135	142	149	155	162	169	176
70	132	139	146	153	160	167	174	181
71	136	143	150	157	165	172	179	186
72	140	147	154	162	169	177	184	191
73	144	151	159	166	174	182	189	197
74	148	155	163	171	179	186	194	202
75	152	160	168	176	184	192	200	208
76	156	164	172	180	189	197	205	213

For BMI above 35, see the National Heart, Lung and Blood Institute site at http://www.nhlbi.nih.gov/guidelines/obesity/bmi_tbl2.htm.

Appendix A

27	28	29	30	31	32	33	34	35
			Body Weight (pounds)					
129	134	138	143	148	153	158	162	167
133	138	143	148	153	158	163	168	173
138	143	148	153	158	163	168	174	179
143	148	153	158	164	169	174	180	185
147	153	158	164	169	175	180	186	191
152	158	163	169	175	180	186	191	197
157	163	169	174	180	186	192	197	204
162	168	174	180	186	192	198	204	210
167	173	179	186	192	198	204	210	216
172	178	185	191	198	204	211	217	223
177	184	190	197	203	210	216	223	230
182	189	196	203	209	216	223	230	236
188	195	202	209	216	222	229	236	243
193	200	208	215	222	229	236	243	250
199	206	213	221	228	235	242	250	258
204	212	219	227	235	242	250	257	265
210	218	225	233	241	249	256	264	272
216	224	232	240	248	256	264	272	279
221	230	238	246	254	263	271	279	287

APPENDIX B

LOW-GLYCEMIC FOODS

Adding these types of foods to your meals will help control levels of glucose in your blood, making it easier for your body to use the food you eat as energy rather than storing it as fat. You don't have to limit your foods to those on the list below, but if you include some of them in each of your meals, the net effect of your meal will be a slower conversion to blood sugar. Eating low-glycemic foods reduces the risk of diabetes and heart disease.

Categories of Foods That Are Low-Glycemic

Proteins, Dairy, and Fats

Red meat and pork (lean cuts are healthier)	Fats (high-quality fats, such as olive oil, are preferred)
Poultry	
Fish	Milk, whole and low-fat
Cheese	Ice cream, regular fat

Vegetables

Artichokes	Cabbage	Corn
Avocado	Carrots	Cucumber
Bok choy	Cauliflower	String beans
Broccoli	Celery	

Fresh Fruit

Apple	Grapefruit	Pear
Apricot	Grapes	Plum
Banana	Mango	Strawberries
Cantaloupe	Orange	
Cherries	Peach	

Appendix B

Grains

Barley	Corn
Buckwheat	Brown rice
Bulgur	

Beans and Legumes

Black-eyed peas	Lima beans
Butter beans	Mung beans
Chickpeas or garbanzo beans	Navy beans
	Pinto beans
Kidney beans	Soybeans

Pasta

Varieties made from durum wheat, whole grains, or egg

Nuts

Cashews	Pecans	Peanuts

Source: Foster-Powell, K, Holt, SH and Brand-Miller, JC, International table of glycemic index and glycemic load values: 2002. *American Journal of Clinical Nutrition* 2002; 76(1): 5–56.

SELECTED REFERENCES

Alesci, S, Manoli, I, Costello, R, et al (eds.). *Carnitine: The Science Behind a Conditionally Essential Nutrient.* New York, NY: New York Academy of Sciences, 2004.

Ames, BN, and Liu, J. "Delaying the mitochondrial decay of aging with acetylcarnitine." *Annals of the New York Academy of Sciences,* 2004; 1033:108–116.

Anand, I, Chandrashekhan, Y, De Giuli, F, et al. "Acute and chronic effects of propionyl-L-carnitine on the hemodynamics, exercise capacity, and hormones in patients with congestive heart failure." *Cardiovascular Drugs and Therapy,* 1998; 12(3):291–299.

Barker, GA, Green, S, Askew, CD, et al. "Effect of propionyl-L-carnitine on exercise performance in peripheral arterial disease." *Medicine and Science in Sports and Exercise,* 2001; 33(9):1415–1422.

Biagiotti, G, and Cavallini, G. "Acetyl-L-carnitine vs tamoxifen in the oral therapy of Peyronie's disease: a preliminary report." *BJU International,* 2001; 88(1): 63–67.

Brass, EP, Adler, S, Sietsema, KE, et al. "Intravenous L-carnitine increases plasma carnitine, reduces fatigue, and may preserve exercise capacity in hemodialysis patients." *American Journal of Kidney Diseases,* 2001; 37(5):1018–1028.

Cacciatore, L, Cerio, R, Ciarimboli, M, et al. "The therapeutic effect of L-carnitine in patients with exercise-induced stable angina: a controlled study." *Drugs Under Experimental and Clinical Research,* 1991; 17(4): 225–235.

Cavallini, G, Caracciolo, S, Vitali, G, et al. "Carnitine versus androgen administration in the treatment of sexual dysfunction, depressed mood, and fatigue

Selected References

associated with male aging." *Urology*, 2004; 63(4): 641–646.

Cerretelli, P, and Marconi, C, "L-carnitine supplementation in humans: the effects on physical performance." *International Journal of Sports Medicine,* 1990; 11:1014.

Cherchi, A, Lai, C, Angelino, F, et al. "Effects of L-carnitine on exercise tolerance in chronic stable angina: a multicenter, double-blind, randomized, placebo controlled crossover study." *International Journal of Clinical Pharmacology, Therapy and Toxicology*, 1985; 23(10):569–572.

De Rosa, M, Boggia, B, Amalfi, B, et al. "Correlation between seminal carnitine and functional spermatozoal characteristics in men with semen dysfunction of various origins." *Drugs in R&D*, 2005; 6(1):1–9.

Feher, J, Kovacs, B, Kovacs, I, et al. "Improvement of visual functions and fundus alterations in early age-related macular degeneration treated with a combination of acetyl-L-carnitine, n-3 fatty acids, and coenzyme Q_{10}. *Ophthalmologica*, 2005; 219(3):154–166.

Garolla, A, Maiorino, M, Roverato, A, et al. "Oral carnitine supplementation increases sperm motility in asthenozoospermic men with normal sperm phospholipid hydroperoxide glutathione peroxidase levels." *Fertility and Sterility*, 2005; 83(2):355–361.

Giancaterini, A, De Gaetano, A, Mingrone, G, et al. "Acetyl-L-carnitine infusion increases glucose disposal in type 2 diabetic patients." *Metabolism*, 2000; 49(6): 704–708.

Hagen, TM, Liu, J, Lykkesfeldt, J, et al. "Feeding acetyl-L-carnitine and lipoic acid to old rats significantly improves metabolic function while decreasing oxidative stress." *Proceedings of the National Academy of Sciences USA*, 2002; 99(4):1870–1875.

Hampton, T. "Study reveals mitochondrial role in aging." *Journal of the American Medical Association*, 2005; 294:672.

Hart, AM, Wilson, AD, Montovani, C, et al. "Acetyl-L-carnitine: a pathogenesis based treatment for HIV-associated antiretroviral toxic neuropathy." *AIDS*, 2004; 18(11):1549–1560.

Hiatt, WR, Regensteiner, JG, Creager, MA, et al. "Propionyl-L-carnitine improves exercise performance and functional status in patients with claudication." *American Journal of Medicine,* 2001; 110(8):616–622.

Iyer, RN, Khan, AA, Gupta, A, et al. "L-carnitine moderately improves the exercise tolerance in chronic stable angina." *The Journal of the Association of Physicians of India,* 2000; 48(11):1050–1052.

Kamikawa, T, Suzuki, Y, Kobayashi, A, et al. "Effects of L-carnitine on exercise tolerance in patients with stable angina pectoris." *Japanese Heart Journal,* 1984; 25(4): 587–597.

Kaats, GR, Wise, JA, Blum, K, et al. "The short-term therapeutic efficacy of treating obesity with a plan of improved nutrition and moderate caloric restriction." *Current Therapeutic Research,* 1992; 51(2):261–274.

Kelly, GS. "Insulin resistance: lifestyle and nutritional interventions." *Alternative Medicine Review,* 2000; 5(2):109–132.

Kraemer, WJ, Volek, JS, French, DN, et al. "The effects of L-carnitine L-tartrate supplementation on hormonal responses to resistance exercise and recovery." *Journal of Strength and Conditioning Research,* 2003;17(3): 455–462.

"L-Carnitine." *Alternative Medicine Review,* 2005; 10 (1):42–50.

Lenzi, A, Sgro, P, Salacone, P, et al. "A placebo-controlled double-blind randomized trial of the use of combined L-carnitine and l-acetyL-carnitine treatment in men with asthenozoospermia." *Fertility and Sterility,* 2004; 81(6):1578–1584.

Leonhardt, M, and Langhans, W. "Fatty acid oxidation and control of food intake." *Physiology and Behavior,* 2004; 83(4):645–651.

Liu, J, Head, E, Gharib, AM, et al. "Memory loss in old rats is associated with brain mitochondrial decay and RNA/DNA oxidation: partial reversal by feeding acetyl-L-carnitine and/or R-alpha-lipoic acid." *Proceedings of the National Academy of Sciences USA,* 2002; 99(4): 2356–2361.

Liu, J, Head, E, Kuratsune, H, et al. "Comparison of

Selected References

the effects of L-carnitine and acetyl-L-carnitine on carnitine levels, ambulatory activity, and oxidative stress biomarkers in the brain of old rats." *Annals of the New York Academy of Sciences*, 2004; 1033:117–131.

Liu, J, Killilea, DW, and Ames, BN. "Age-associated mitochondrial oxidative decay: improvement of carnitine acetyltransferase substrate-binding affinity and activity in brain by feeding old rats acetyl-L-carnitine and/or R-alpha -lipoic acid." *Proceedings of the National Academy of Sciences USA*, 2002; 99(4):1876–1881.

Luppa, D, and Loster, H. "L-carnitine through urine and sweat and athletes in dependence on energy expenditure during training." In: *Carnitine—Pathobiochemical Basics and Clinical Applications*. Bochum, Germany: Ponte Press, 1996, pp. 278–279.

Lurz, R, and Fischer, R. [translation] "Carnitine as supporting agent in weight loss in adiposity." *Medical Journal for Natural Therapy*, 1998; 39(1):12–15.

Maestri, A, De Pasquale Ceratti, A, Cundari, S, et al. "A pilot study on the effect of acetyl-L-carnitine in paclitaxel- and cisplatin-induced peripheral neuropathy." *Tumori*, 2005; 91(2):135–138.

McCarty, MF. "The unique merits of a low-fat diet for weight control." *Medical Hypotheses*, 1986; 20(2):183–197.

Montgomery, SA, Thal, LJ, Amrein, R. "Meta-analysis of double blind randomized controlled clinical trials of acetyl-L-carnitine versus placebo in the treatment of mild cognitive impairment and mild Alzheimer's disease." *International Clinical Psychopharmacology*, 2003; 18(2):61–71.

Pauly, DF, and Pepine, CJ. "Ischemic heart disease: metabolic approaches to management." *Clinical Cardiology*, 2004; 27:439–441.

Reda, E, D'Iddio, S, Nicolai, R, et al. "The carnitine system and body composition." *Acta Diabetologica*, 2003; 40 (Suppl) 1:S106–113.

Sima, AA, Calvani, M, Mehra, M, et al. "Acetyl-L-carnitine improves pain, nerve regeneration, and vibratory perception in patients with chronic diabetic neuropathy: an analysis of two randomized placebo-controlled trials." *Diabetes Care*, 2005; 28(1):89–94.

Tomassini, V, Pozzilli, C, Onesti, E, et al. "Comparison of the effects of acetyl-L-carnitine and amantadine for the treatment of fatigue in multiple sclerosis: results of a pilot, randomised, double-blind, crossover trial." *Journal of Neurological Sciences*, 2004; 218(1–2):103–108.

Vermeulen, RC, and Scholte, HR. "Exploratory open label, randomized study of acetyl- and propionyl carnitine in chronic fatigue syndrome." *Psychosomatic Medicine*, 2004; 66(2):276–282.

Volek, JS, Kraemer, WJ, Rubin, MR, et al. "L-carnitine L-tartrate supplementation favorably affects markers of recovery from exercise stress." *American Journal of Physiology Endocrinology and Metabolism*, 2002; 282(2):E474–482.

Wutzke, KD, and Lorenz, H. "The effect of L-carnitine on fat oxidation, protein turnover, and body composition in slightly overweight subjects." *Metabolism*, 2004; 53(8):1002–1006.

OTHER BOOKS AND RESOURCES

GreatLife Magazine
Consumer magazine with articles on vitamins, minerals, herbs, and foods.
Available for free at many health and natural food stores.

Let's Live Magazine
Consumer magazine with emphasis on the health benefits of vitamins, minerals, and herbs.
Customer service:
1-800-676-4333
P.O. Box 74908
Los Angeles, CA 90004
Subscriptions: 12 issues per year, $19.95 in the U.S.; $31.95 outside the U.S.

Physical Magazine
Magazine oriented to body builders and other serious athletes.
Customer service:
1-800-676-4333
P.O. Box 74908
Los Angeles, CA 90004
Subscriptions: 12 issues per year, $19.95 in the U.S.; $31.95 outside the U.S.

The Nutrition Reporter™ newsletter
Monthly newsletter that summarizes recent medical research on vitamins, minerals, and herbs.
Customer service:
P.O. Box 30246
Tucson, AZ 85751-0246

e-mail: jack@thenutritionreporter.com
www.nutritionreporter.com
Subscriptions: $26 per year (12 issues) in the U.S.; $32 U.S. or $48 CNC for Canada; $38 for other countries

INDEX

Acetyl-L-carnitine (ALC), 1–2, 3–9, 58–62, 63–66, 70–72, 73
Acta Diabetologica, 57
Adenosine triphosphate. *See* ATP.
Aerobic exercise, 27
Aging, 3, 27–41, 58–62, 68–69, 71
 disease and, 60–62
 exercise and, 27–41
AIDS, 61
ALA. *See* Alpha lipoic acid.
ALCAR, 60, 61
Alpha lipoic acid, 71
Alzheimer's disease, 4, 5, 30, 60
American College of Cardiology, 12
American College of Sports Medicine, 27
American Diabetes Association, 63
American Heart Association, 12, 13, 27
American Journal of Clinical Nutrition, 47, 50
American Journal of Kidney Diseases, 32
American Journal of Medicine, 32
American Journal of Physiology Endocrinology and Metabolism, 34
Ames, Bruce, 58–60

Amino acids, 38–39
AmminoCarnitines, 6, 38, 38–39, 70–71, 73
Angina pectoris, 3, 11
Antioxidants, 47
Appetite, 46
Appetite control strategies, 50–51
Arrhythmia, 11–12
Arteriosclerosis, 10
Ascorbic acid. *See* Vitamin C.
Atherosclerosis, 10
ATP, 18, 20–23, 40, 53

Back pain, 30
Baltimore Longitudinal Study of Aging, 27
Baylor College of Medicine, 46
Beans, 79
Biochemical and Biophysical Research Communications, 18
BJU International, 69
Blood-brain barrier, 5–6
Blood sugar. *See* Glucose.
Bloomer, Richard, 38–39, 41
Body mass index (BMI), 45, 51, 75–77
Bone density, 30
Bone mass, 29
Brain health, 71
Breakfast, 50

Calories, 43

Cancer, 61–62
Carbohydrates, 48–50
Cardiomyopathy, 11
Cardiovascular Drugs and Therapy, 16, 19
Carnitine. See L-carnitine.
Carnitine: Pathobiochemical Basics and Clinical Applications, 34
Carnitine: The Science Behind a Conditionally Essential Nutrient, 8, 59
Cellular health, 4
Children, 4
Children's Hospital Oakland Research Institute, 58
Cholesterol, 39
Chromium, 71
Chronic fatigue syndrome (CFS), 4, 61
Circulation, 27
Clinical Cardiology, 13, 20
Clinical Investigator, 19
Coenyzme Q_{10}. See CoQ_{10}.
Columbia University, 51
Congestive heart failure. See Heart failure.
CoQ_{10}, 17–20, 22–23, 61, 71
  studies, 18–20
  synergy with L-carnitine, 17–20
C-reactive protein. See CRP.
CRP, 29
Current Atherosclerosis Reports, 46

Dairy products, 3, 43, 78
Depression, 30
Diabetes, 7, 63–66, 71
  preventing, 65–66
Diabetes Care, 64
Dialysis, 5
Diastolic function, 20

Diet, 46–52, 70. See also Food.
DNA, 59
D-Ribose, 20–23, 71
  synergy with CoQ_{10}, 20–23
Drugs Under Experimental and Clinical Research, 16
Drugs R&D, 68
Duke University Medical Center, 26

East Virginia Medical School, 51
Endothelium, 40
Energy, 26–41
Ester Carnitine, 6, 39, 41, 61, 71–72, 73
European Journal of Heart Failure, 21
Exercise, 7, 9, 15, 26–41, 66, 70
  overcoming excuses to, 31
  starting a program, 36–38

Fat, 66
Fat burning, 52–53
Fatigue, exercise-related, 4
Fats, 47–48, 66, 78
Fertility, male, 67–69, 71
Fertility and Sterility, 67
Fiber, 66
Fibromyalgia, 4
Fish oil, 71
Fitness, 26–41
Fleg, Jerome, 28
Flour, 66
Food, 46–53
  low-glycemic, 78–79
  See also Diet.
Free radicals, 25
Fruits, 47, 78

Gangwisch, James, 51

Index

Glucose, 49–50, 65–66
Glycemic foods, low, 78–79
Glycemic index, 49, 78–79
Glycemic load, 50, 66
Glycogen, 40
GPLC. *See* Ester Carnitine.
Grains, 79

Hagan, Tory, 58–59
Harbor University of California, 32, 54
Heart, 10–25, 70
   conditions, 10–13
   CoQ_{10} and, 18–20
   preventing problems, 23–24
   transplants, 18–19
Heart attack, 3
   surviving, 14
Heart disease and quality of life, 14–17
Heart failure, 3, 12, 13–14, 15–20
High-density lipoprotein (HDL). *See* Cholesterol.
HIV, 61

Idiopathic, 13
Inflammation, 29
Insulin, 49, 57, 63, 66
Insulin resistance, 4, 65–66
   lifestyle factors and, 66
Intermittent claudication, 4, 31–32
International Journal of Clinical Pharmacology, Therapy and Toxicology, 15
International Journal of Sports Medicine, 33
Iron, 3
Ischemia, 11, 21

Jalali, Rehan, 33

Japanese Heart Journal, 15
Journal of Neurological Sciences, 61
Journal of Strength and Conditioning Research, 34
Journal of the American Dietetic Association, 45
Journal of the Association of Physicians of India, 17
Journal of the American Medical Association, 59

Kidney disease, 32–33

Lancet, 21
L-carnitine, 1–2, 3–9, 10–25, 26–41, 42–57, 58–62, 63–66, 67–69, 70–72, 73–74
   CoQ_{10} and, 17–20
   deficiencies, 4
   diabetes and, 63–66
   dosages, 70–71
   d-ribose and, 20–23
   exercise and, 26–41
   fat and, 52–53
   food sources of, 7
   forms, 5–6, 38–39, 70–71
   heart health and, 10–25
   male fetility and, 67–69
   nerve damage and, 64–65
   program, 70–72
   safety, 8
   studies, 15–17, 54–57
   supplement benefits, 8–9
   supplement needs, 6–8
   weight loss and, 42–57
Legumes, 79

Lifestyle, 66, 70
Lipids, 39
Lipoic acid. See Alpha lipoic acid.
Low-density lipoprotein (LDL). See Cholesterol.
Low-glycemic, 50
L-tartrate, 6
Lysine, 3

Macular degeneration, 61
Magnesium, 71
Meat, 2, 3
Medical Hypotheses, 56
Medical Journal for Natural Therapy, 57
Medicine and Science in Sports and Exercise, 31
Men and aging, 68–69
Metabolic cardiology, 22–23
Metabolism, 54, 65
Methionine, 3
Milk products. See Dairy products.
Mitochondria, 4, 60, 67–69
Molecular and Cellular Biochemistry, 19
Multiple sclerosis (MS), 61
Muscle weakness, 4
Mycocardial infarction, 11
Myocardial ischemia, 11

National Center for Complementary and Alternative Medicine, 8
National Institute of Child Health and Human Development, 8
National Institute of Mental Health, 8
National Institutes of Health. See U.S. National Institutes of Health.
National Weight Control Registry, 52
Nervous sytem, 63–65
Neuropathy, diabetic, 4, 63–66
New England Journal of Medicine, 26
Niacin. See Vitamin B_3.
North American Association for the Study of Obersity, 51
Nutrition, 35
Nutrition. See Diet.
Nuts, 79

Office of Dietary Supplements, 8, 59
Omega-3 fatty acids, 61, 66
Ophthalmologica, 61
Osteoporosis, 29
Oxidation, 40
Oxygen, 27, 40

Parkinson's disease, 4
Pasta, 79
Peripheral arterial disease, 31–32
Peyronie's disease, 69,
Physician's Committee for Responsible Medicine, 42, 43
Physiology and Behavior, 46
Prediabetes, 63–66
Propionyl-L-carnitine (PLC), 5–6, 31, 38–41
exercise and, 39–41
Prostate, 68
Protein, 47, 66, 78
ProXeed, 71
Psychosomatic Medicine, 61
Pyridoxine. See Vitamin B_6.

Index

Resistance training, 29
Resting metabolic rate (RMR), 55–56
Ribose. *See* D-Ribose.

Sex life, 30
Sigma-tau Health-Science, 38
Simontacchi, Carol, 42
Sinatra, Stephen, 20, 22–23, 24, 60
Sinatra Solution, The, 22
Six-Pack Diet Plan, 33
Sleep, 51
Sperm motility, 67–69
Sugar, 66
Syndrome X, 49
Systolic function, 21

Testosterone, 68–69
Triglycerides, 39
Tumori: A Journal of Experimental and Clinical Oncology, 61–62

University of California, Berkeley, 58
University of Colorado Health Sciences Center, 31
University of Connecticut, Storrs, 34
University of Florida College of Medicine, 13
University of Memphis, 38–39
University of Texas, San Antonio, 54
University of Washington School of Medicine, 47
Urology, 68
U.S. Agency for Healthcare Research and Quality, 10
U.S. Centers for Disease Control and Prevention, 27, 30
U.S. National Heart, Lung, and Blood Institutes, 28
U.S. National Institutes of Health, 8, 59

Vanadyl sulfate, 71
Vegetables, 47, 66, 78
Vegetarian diet deficiencies, 4, 6
Veteran's Administration Medical Center, Minneapolis, 16
Vitamin B_3, 3
Vitamin B_6, 3
Vitamin C, 3
VO2, 27

Wayne State University, 64
Weight gain, 66
Weight loss, 9, 42–57, 70
 basics, 52
 studies, 53–57
Weight Success for a Lifetime, 52
Weight training, 29–30, 40